Recurrence of the Disease in the Renal Graft

John Libbey Eurotext
127, avenue de la République
92120 Montrouge
Tél.: 33 (0) 1 46 73 06 60
e-mail: contact@john-libbey-eurotext.fr
http://www.john-libbey-eurotext.fr

John Libbey and Company Ltd
Collier House,
163-169 Brompton Road, Knightsbridge
London SW3 1 PY, England
Tel.: 44 (0) 20 75 81 24 49

CIC Edizioni Internazionali
Corso Trieste 42
00198 Roma, Italia
Tel.: 39 06 841 26 73

© John Libbey Eurotext, 2001
ISBN: 2-7420-0414-9

Illustration de couverture
© Twice Daily, 2001

All rights reserved. No part of this publication may be reproduced without written permission from the Publisher or the Centre Français du Copyright, 20, rue des Grands-Augustins, 75006 Paris.

Recurrence of the Disease in the Renal Graft

33rd International Conference
on Transplantation
and Clinical Immunology

CITIC 2001
29, 30 November 2001

Edited by
Pierre Cochat

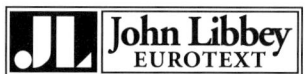

Organizing Committee

P. Cochat

J.-M. Dubernard

J. Traeger

J.-L. Touraine

J.-P. Revillard

C. Dupuy

J.-L. Colpart

V. Lachat

X. Martin

O. Bastien

D. Guillot

International Advisory Committee CITIC

D. Forti *(Milano)*

M. Goldman *(Brussels)*

G.N. Grinyo *(Barcelona)*

P. Lang *(Paris)*

P.J. Morris *(Oxford)*

G. Opelz *(Heidelberg)*

G. Segoloni *(Torino)*

Contents

Tribute to Charles Mérieux
J. Traeger XI

Nephrotic syndrome

Influence of recurrence on graft and patient survival
J.D. Briggs 1

"Recurrent noncompliance": the behavioral pitfall for long-term successful outcome in end-stage renal disease
S. De Geest, F. Dobbels, I. Cleemput, M. Fliedner, J. Steiger, D. Manhaeve, Y. Vanrenterghem 7

Predicting the natural course of nephrotic syndrome in children. An integrate clinical and molecular approach
G.M. Ghiggeri, F. Perfumo 15

Recurrence of focal and segmental glomerulosclerosis in renal transplant: clinical and pathological features
D. Droz, D. Anglicheau, C. Legendre 23

Podocyte injury underlies progression of chronic renal disease. Evidence from experimental models
W. Kriz 27

Post-transplant proteinuria in Finnish type nephrotic syndrome
C. Holmberg, J. Patrakka, J. Laine, H. Jalanko 35

Intragraft events in post-transplant recurrent nephrotic syndrome
A.D. Schachter 39

Circulating mediators of proteinuria in nephrotic syndrome
E.H. Garin 45

A practical approach to the prediction of recurrence of focal segmental glomerulosclerosis in renal allograft recipients
N.J.A. Webb 51

Plasma treatments for patients with recurrence of focal segmental glomerular sclerosis after renal transplantation
D. Hristea, L. Le Berre, C. Guyot, M. Hourmant, J.-P. Soulillou, J. Dantal 57

Other diseases

Recurrence of the disease in the renal graft: diabetic nephropathy
P. Petruzzo, N. Lefrançois, L. Badet, I. Desormais, J.-M. Dubernard, X. Martin. 67

Renal transplantation in patients with systemic lupus erythematosus
P. Grimbert, E. Thervet 75

Recurrence of ANCA-associated glomerulonephritis after successful renal transplantation
L. Rostaing 79

Strategies to avoid recurrence of oxalosis in the renal allograft
B. Hoppe, E. Leumann 81

Recurrence of membranoproliferative glomerulonephritis after renal transplantation
R. Cahen 89

Recurrent membranous nephropathy after kidney transplantation
C. Pouteil-Noble 97

Recurrent IgA nephropathy after kidney transplantation
J. Floege 107

Recurrent and *de novo* anti-GBM disease in the kidney graft
Y. Pirson, E. Goffin, J.-P. Cosyns, L.-H. Noel, J.-P. Squifflet 111

De novo renal diseases after renal transplantation
S. Hariharan 117

Recurrent disease in the urological patient following renal transplantation
G.H. Neild, C.R.J. Woodhouse, S. Wood, R. Nauth-Misir, S. Nathan, N. Jenkins. 123

Contributors

Anglicheau D., Service de Néphrologie, Hôpital Saint-Louis, 1, avenue Cl.-Vellefaux, 75010 Paris, France.

Badet L., Service d'Urologie et Chirurgie de la Transplantation, Hôpital Édouard-Herriot, 5, place d'Arsonval, 69437 Lyon Cedex 3, France.

Briggs J.D., ERA-EDTA Registry, Academic Medical Centre, University of Amsterdam, The Netherlands.

Cahen R., Service de Néphrologie, Centre Hospitalier Lyon-Sud, 165, chemin Grand-Revoyet, 69495 Pierre-Bénite Cedex, France.

Cleemput I., Institute of Nursing Science, University of Basel, Bernoullistrassse 28, CH 4056 Basel, Switzerland.

Cosyns J.-P., Service de Pathologie, Cliniques Universitaires Saint-Luc, 10, avenue Hippocrate, B-120 Brussels, Belgium.

Dantal J., ITERT-INSERM U437, CHU, Hôtel-Dieu, 30, boulevard Jean-Monnet, 44093 Nantes Cedex 01, France.

De Geest S., Institute of Nursing Science, University of Basel, Bernoullistrassse 28, CH 4003 Basel, Switzerland.

Desormais I., Service d'Urologie et Chirurgie de la Transplantation, Hôpital Édouard-Herriot, 5, place d'Arsonval, 69437 Lyon Cedex 3, France.

Dobbels F., Institute of Nursing Science, University of Basel, Bernoullistrassse 28, CH 4056 Basel, Switzerland.

Droz D., Service d'Anatomie Pathologique, Hôpital Saint-Louis, 1, avenue Cl.-Vellefaux, 75010 Paris, France.

Dubernard J.-M., Service d'Urologie et Chirurgie de la Transplantation, Hôpital Édouard-Herriot, 5, place d'Arsonval, 69437 Lyon Cedex 3, France.

Fliedner M., Institute of Nursing Science, University of Basel, Bernoullistrassse 28, CH 4056 Basel, Switzerland.

Floege J., Division of Nephrology, Medizinische Klinik II, RWTH Aachen, 52057 Aachen, Germany.

Garin E.H., USF Pediatric Nephrology, 17 Davis Blvd, 2nd Floor, Tampa FL 33606, USA.

Ghiggeri G.M., U.O. Nefrologia Instituto G. Gaslini, Largo G. Gaslini 5, 16148 Genova, Italy.

Goffin E., Service de Néphrologie, Cliniques Universitaires Saint-Luc, 10, avenue Hippocrate, B-120 Brussels, Belgium.

Grimbert P., Service de Néphrologie, Hôpital Henri-Mondor, 51, avenue du Maréchal-de-Lattre-de-Tassigny, 94010 Créteil, France.

Guyot C., ITERT-INSERM U437, CHU, Hôtel-Dieu, 30, boulevard Jean-Monnet, 44093 Nantes Cedex 01, France.

Hariharan S., Medical College of Wisconsin, Division of Nephrology, 9200 West Wisconsin Avenue, Milwaukee, Wi 53226, USA.

Holmberg C., Hospital for Children and Adolescents, University of Helsinki, 00290, Helsinki, Finland.

Hoppe B., Division of Pediatric Nephrology, University Children's Hospital Cologne, Josef-Stelzmann Str. 9, D-50924 Cologne, Germany.

Hourmant M., ITERT-INSERM U437, CHU, Hôtel-Dieu, 30, boulevard Jean-Monnet, 44093 Nantes Cedex 01, France.

Hristrea D., ITERT-INSERM U437, CHU, Hôtel-Dieu, 30, boulevard Jean-Monnet, 44093 Nantes Cedex 01, France.

Jalanko H., Hospital for Children and Adolescents, University of Helsinki, 00290, Helsinki, Finland.

Jenkins N., Institute of Urology and Nephrology, University College London and Renal Unit, UCL Hospitals, London W1N 8AA, United Kingdom.

Kriz W., Institut für Anatomie und Zellbiologie, Universität Heidelberg, Im Neuenheimer Feld 307, 69120 Heidelberg, Germany.

Laine J., Hospital for Children and Adolescents, University of Helsinki, 00290, Helsinki, Finland.

Le Berre L., ITERT-INSERM U437, CHU, Hôtel-Dieu, 30, boulevard Jean-Monnet, 44093 Nantes Cedex 01, France.

Lefrançois N., Service d'Urologie et Chirurgie de la Transplantation, Hôpital Édouard-Herriot, 5, place d'Arsonval, 69437 Lyon Cedex 3, France.

Legendre C., Service de Néphrologie, Hôpital Saint-Louis, 1, avenue Cl.-Vellefaux, 75010 Paris, France.

Leumann E., University Children's Hospital Zurich, Switzerland.

Manhaeve D., Epsilon Group, Bedrijvencentrum Industriepark Haasrode, Interleuvenlaan 62, B-3001, Leuven, Belgium.

Martin X., Service d'Urologie et Chirurgie de la Transplantation, Hôpital Édouard-Herriot, 5, place d'Arsonval, 69437 Lyon Cedex 3, France.

Nathan S., Institute of Urology and Nephrology, University College London and Renal Unit, UCL Hospitals, London W1N 8AA, United Kingdom.

Nauth-Misir R., Institute of Urology and Nephrology, University College London and Renal Unit, UCL Hospitals, London W1N 8AA, United Kingdom.

Neild G.H., Institute of Urology and Nephrology, University College, Middlesex Hospital, Mortimer Street, London W1N 8AA, United Kingdom.

Noel L.-H., Service de Pathologie, Hôpital Necker, Paris, France.

Patrakka J., Hospital for Children and Adolescents, University of Helsinki, 00290, Helsinki, Finland.

Perfumo F., U.O. Nefrologia Instituto G. Gaslini, Largo G. Gaslini 5, 16148 Genova, Italy.

Petruzzo P., Service d'Urologie et Chirurgie de la Transplantation, Hôpital Édouard-Herriot, 5, place d'Arsonval, 69437 Lyon Cedex 3, France.

Pirson Y., Service de Néphrologie, Cliniques Universitaires Saint-Luc, 10, avenue Hippocrate, B-120 Brussels, Belgium.

Pouteil-Noble C., Transplantation and Nephrology Unit, Centre Hospitalier Lyon-Sud, 165, chemin Grand-Revoyet, 69495 Pierre-Bénite Cedex, France, and UFR Lyon-Sud, Université Claude-Bernard.

Rostaing L., Service de Néphrologie-Transplantation, CHU Rangueil, 1, avenue Jean-Pouilhès, 31403 Toulouse Cedex 4, France.

Schachter A.D., Renal Transplant Office, FA-403, Children's Hospital, 300 Longwood Avenue, Boston, MA 02115, USA.

Soulillou J.-P., ITERT-INSERM U437, CHU, Hôtel-Dieu, 30, boulevard Jean-Monnet, 44093 Nantes Cedex 01, France.

Squifflet J.-P., Service de Transplantation rénale, Cliniques Universitaires Saint-Luc, 10, avenue Hippocrate, B-120 Brussels, Belgium.

Steiger J., Department of Transplantation, Immunology and Nephrology, Kantonspital Basel, Petersgrabern 4/6, CH 4031 Basel, Switzerland.

Thervet E., Service de Néphrologie, Hôpital Henri-Mondor, 51, avenue du Maréchal-de-Lattre-de-Tassigny, 94010 Créteil, France.

Vanrenterghem Y., Department of Nephrology, University Hospital of Leuven, Heresstrat 49, B-3000 Leuven, Belgium.

Webb N.J.A., Royal Manchester Children's Hospital, Manchester M 27 4HA, United Kingdom.

Wood S., Institute of Urology and Nephrology, University College London and Renal Unit, UCL Hospitals, London W1N 8AA, United Kingdom.

Woodhouse C.R.J., Institute of Urology and Nephrology, University College London and Renal Unit, UCL Hospitals, London W1N 8AA, United Kingdom.

Recurrence of the Disease in the Renal Graft
Cochat P, ed.
© John Libbey Eurotext, Paris, 2001

Tribute to Charles Mérieux

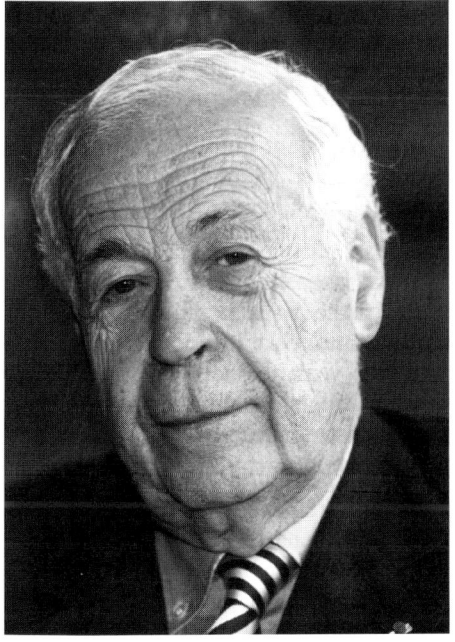

The disappearance of Charles Mérieux marks the close of an exceptionally productive period in the development of human biology; a period where a profound humanitarian mission was backed by a major industrial enterprise.

Charles Mérieux was a true visionary with an extraordinary lucidity in his choices for the future. He knew how to grasp the opportune moment and, after a rapid decision, to move forward decisively. He would then employ patience and tenacity to develop novel ideas and, once his choice was made, he would proceed with calm energy and remarkable perseverance until the success of his project was assured.

This strength of will was backed by a large industrial empire which he had himself built on the basis of the biological laboratory founded by his father, Marcel Mérieux. He had the ability to use the enormous means at his disposal to promote his scientific and humanitarian mission. In 1967 he created the Marcel Mérieux Foundation which supported and promoted numerous projects, meetings, colloquia and symposia, and underwrote research projects and many other activities which sprang from his fertile mind. The many volumes of reports on these activities constitute an exceptionally rich collection.

In this context, Charles Mérieux gave us his unconditional support for the development of the CITIC.

In 1966 we had developed a new type of antilymphocyte serum. With Dr Fries, we had envisaged the use of human thoracic duct lymphocytes as a source of antigen. This material of exceptional purity allowed Dr Carraz of the Lyon Pasteur Institute to immunise his horses under optimal conditions, and to obtain sera with excellent immunosuppressive power and without measurable toxicity. Charles Mérieux immediately suggested that mycophenolate mofetil might have a beneficial effect but there is as yet no evidence to support this. The only available evidence relates to non-specific measures in that a small scale study has shown a beneficial effect of an ACE inhibitor on blood pressure and proteinuria [6].

Focal segmental glomerulosclerosis (FSGS)

The most frequently quoted incidence figure for recurrence of FSGS is 20-30% and this is supported by the figure of 20.5% published in 1992 from the North American Pediatric Renal Transplant Cooperative Study (NAPRTCS) [7]. There are a number of factors which influence the incidence, one of which is age and most of the figures in the literature are from a predominantly paediatric population. If one compares children and adults in the same series, the incidence in children is much higher. In a study from Guy's Hospital, the recurrence rate in children was 50% and in adolescents and adults 11% [8]. A higher recurrence rate has also been found in patients with shorter time intervals between the onset of the native kidney disease and development of renal failure [9]. It has been suggested that live donor kidneys are more prone to recurrent FSGS than those of cadaver origin but there is no good evidence of this. However, it has been reported that the usual survival advantage conferred by a live donor kidney is reduced in the setting of recurrent disease [10]. As this study suggests that there is still some survival advantage from the use of a live donor and as the live donor kidney confers other advantages, it remains a good option for a primary transplant in FSGS patients. The much higher recurrence rate in retransplants where the first has failed from recurrence would argue against the use of a live donor kidney for a retransplant. If one looks at all failed grafts, the percentage being lost as a consequence of recurrent disease was found to be higher for FSGS – in the paediatric age group – than for other types of recurrent disease, the figure in the ERA-EDTA Registry analysis being 24% [1]. Also FSGS usually leads to early failure with only 35% of affected grafts functioning at 2 years [1]. Finally in contrast to most other types of recurrent disease, there is a reasonable prospect of inducing remission of the recurrence by means of plasmapheresis. This can either be used at the time of relapse [11] or carried out immediately prior to the transplant, followed by a further course should there be a recurrence despite prophylactic plasmapheresis [12].

Henoch Schonlein nephritis

This shares a number of features with IgA nephropathy and the pattern of recurrent disease is similar. The most comprehensive report is that of Meulders *et al.* who found a recurrence rate of 35% and graft loss of 11% at 5 years [13].

Other primary nephropathies

Most reports of recurrent membranous nephropathy have come from case reports or small series. The largest series is that of Cosyns *et al.* and this contained 30 cases [14]. The recurrence rate reached 29% after 3 years of follow-up and recurrence had a markedly adverse effect on graft survival with a graft loss of 38% and 52% at 5 and 10 years respectively.

One of the larger series documented recurrent type I MPGN in 33% of cases and this would seem to be a typical figure [15]. While the course of recurrent type I MPGN could not be described as benign, it usually has minimal effect on graft survival over the first 3-5 years as shown by a 2 year survival in an ERA-EDTA analysis of 86% [1].

Type II MPGN is an uncommon condition, hence there is limited experience of recurrent disease. However the incidence of recurrence is undoubtedly high with published figures of up to 100%. Also the ERA-EDTA Registry reported only 43% of affected grafts functioning at 2 years, so recurrence is an important cause of graft loss [1].

Haemolytic uraemic syndrome (HUS)

There are two types, sporadic and epidemic, and recurrence is more likely with the former type. Other predisposing factors to recurrence are older age, the use of calcineurin inhibitors, the use of live donor kidneys and a short time interval between onset of the disease and the time of reaching dialysis dependency [16]. Recurrence of HUS has a markedly adverse effect on graft survival with one year survival of 33.3% in those with recurrence and 76.6% in those without [16]. The use of live donors should probably be avoided in patients with the sporadic type because of the risk of recurrence. Also while it is reasonable to use a calcineurin inhibitor for a first transplant, should a graft fail due to recurrence, this group of drugs should be avoided at the time of a second transplant.

References

1. Briggs JD, Jones E. Recurrence of glomerulonephritis following renal transplantation. *Nephrol Dial Transplant* 1999; 14: 564-5.
2. Hariharan S, Adams MB, Brennan DC, Davis CL, First MR, Johnson CP, Ouseph R, Peddi VR, Pelz CJ, Roza AM, Vincenti F, George V. Recurrent and *de novo* glomerular disease after renal transplantation. *Transplantation* 1999; 68: 635-41.
3. Ohmacht C, Kliem V, Burg M, Nashan B, Schlitt HJ, Brunkhorst R, Koch KM, Floege J. Recurrent immunoglobulin A nephropathy after renal transplantation. *Transplantation* 1997; 64: 1493-6.
4. Lim EC, Terasaki PI. High survival rate of kidney transplants in IgA nephropathy patients. *Clin Transplant* 1992; 6: 100-5.
5. Odum J, Peh CA, Clarkson AR, Bannister KM, Seymour AE, Gillis D, Thomas AC, Mathew TH, Woodroffe AJ. Recurrent mesangial IgA nephritis following renal transplantation. *Nephrol Dial Transplant* 1994; 9: 309-12.
6. Oka K, Imai E, Moriyama T, Akagi Y, Ando A, Hori M, Okuyama O, Toki K, Kyo M, Kokado Y, Takahara S. A clinicopathological study of IgA nephropathy in renal transplant recipients: beneficial effect of angiotensin-converting enzyme inhibitor. *Nephrol Dial Transplant* 2000; 15: 689-95.
7. Tejani A, Stablein DH. Recurrence of focal segmental glomerulosclerosis post transplantation: a special report of the North American pediatric renal transplant cooperative study. *J Am Soc Nephrol* 1992; 2 (Suppl. 3): S258-61.
8. Senggutuvan P, Cameron JS, Hartley RB, Rigden S, Chantler C, Haycock G, Williams DG, Ogg C, Koffman G. Recurrence of focal segmental glomerulosclerosis in transplanted kidneys: analysis of incidence and risk factors in 59 allografts. *Pediatr Nephrol* 1990; 4: 21-8.

9. Ramos EL, Tisher CC. Recurrent diseases in the kidney transplant. *Am J Kidney Dis* 1994; 24: 142-54.
10. Baum MA, Stablein DM, Panzarino VM, Tejani A, Harmon WE, Alexander SR. Loss of living donor renal allograft survival advantage in children with focal segmental glomerulosclerosis. *Kidney Int* 2001; 59: 328-33.
11. Andresdottir MB, Ajubi N, Croockewit S, Assmann KJM, Hilbrands LB, Wetzels JFM. Recurrent focal glomerulosclerosis: natural course and treatment with plasma exchange. *Nephrol Dial Transplant* 1999; 14: 2650-6.
12. Ohta T, Kawaguchi H, Hattori M, Komatsu Y, Akioka Y, Nagata M, Shiraga H, Ito K, Takahashi K, Ishikawa N, Tanabe K, Yamaguchi Y, Ota K. Effect of pre and postoperative plasmapheresis on post-transplant recurrence of focal segmental glomerulosclerosis in children. *Transplantation* 2001; 71: 628-33.
13. Meulders Q, Pirson Y, Cosyns JP, Squifflet JP, van Ypersele de Strihou C. Course of Henoch-Schonlein nephritis after renal transplantation. *Transplantation* 1994; 58: 1179-86.
14. Cosyns JP, Couchoud C, Pouteil-Noble C, Squifflet JP, Pirson Y. Recurrence of membranous nephropathy after renal transplantation: probability, outcome and risk factors. *Clin Nephrol* 1998; 50: 144-53.
15. Andresdottir MB, Assmann KJM, Hoitsma AJ, Koene RAP, Wetzels JFM. Recurrence of type I membranoproliferative glomerulonephritis after renal transplantation. *Transplantation* 1997; 63: 1628-33.
16. Ducloux D, Rebibou JM, Semhoun-Ducloux S, Jamali M, Fournier V, Bresson-Vautrin C, Chalopin JM. Recurrence of hemolytic-uremic syndrome in renal transplant recipients. *Transplantation* 1998; 65: 1405-7.

"Recurrent noncompliance":
the behavioral pitfall for long-term successful outcome in end-stage renal disease

Sabina De Geest[1,2], Fabienne Dobbels[1], Irina Cleemput[1], Monica Fliedner[1], Jürg Steiger[3], Dominique Manhaeve[4], Yves Vanrenterghem[5]

[1] Institute of Nursing Science, Switzerland
[2] Center for Health Services and Nursing Research, School of Public Health, Leuven, Belgium
[3] Department of Transplantation, Immunology and Nephrology, Kantonsspital Basel, Switzerland
[4] Epsilon Group, Bedrijvencentrum Industriepark Haasrode, Leuven, Belgium
[5] Department of Nephrology, University Hospital of Leuven, Belgium

Noncompliance with the therapeutic regimen is recognized as a major issue in patients with end stage renal disease as it jeopardizes the effectiveness of the prescribed treatment regimen and as it is associated with increased health care costs. This paper addresses the issue of "recurrent noncompliance" in patients with end stage renal disease including both patients on dialysis as well as transplant recipients. More specifically, the predictive value of noncompliance occurring during different phases of end stage renal disease for subsequent noncompliance and clinical outcome will be reviewed. Time on dialysis, the time after transplantation and, in unfavorable circumstances, return to dialysis and retransplantation are the three time periods that will be taken into consideration. This timeline creates a relevant framework to organize the compliance literature and to explore the unique contribution of the behavioral dimension on outcomes in the management of patients with end stage renal disease. Special attention will be given to noncompliance with immunosuppressive drugs after renal transplantation. Please note that this review focuses only on behavioral factors as predictors of future behavior and clinical outcomes. It does not include studies that assess the impact of psychosocial risk factors such as psychiatric diagnoses or substance abuse on compliance and clinical outcomes.

Dialysis noncompliance as a predictor for post-transplant noncompliance and clinical outcome

The dialysis regimen consists of four major aspects, namely, following dietary and medication guidelines, adherence to fluid restrictions and attendance to the dialysis sessions. Noncompliance with the dialysis regimen is substantial, ranging from 20% to 80% for various parts of the dialysis regimen [1-6]. The Best Practice Guidelines for Renal Transplantation state that "... psychological evaluation of transplant candidates may be useful in assessing compliance with future immunosuppressive treatment" [7].

This evaluation also implies a behavioral assessment in view of noncompliance with the dialysis regimen as a predictor for future post-transplant compliance.

Transplant clinicians perceive dialysis noncompliance to be a reliable predictor of post-transplant noncompliance [8-10]. Ramos *et al.* [8] assessed viewpoints of 182 transplant centers and showed that 83% stated (response rate 81%) that dialysis attendance rates were an important indicator of adherence after transplantation. A nearly similar rate of 77% of the transplant health care workers, questioned in an international study, perceived pretransplant noncompliance to be an important predictor of post-transplant noncompliance [9]. A recent national random survey among US nephrologists asked these nephrologists if patients should be referred for transplantation based on hypothetical patient scenarios. A history of noncompliance was associated with low rates of recommendation for transplantation [10].

It is not unexpected that a relationship between noncompliance with the dialysis regimen and noncompliance post-transplant is hypothesized as there is strong evidence from other chronic patient populations showing that past noncompliance behavior is the best predictor for current and future noncompliance behavior [11]. Yet, very scarce empirical evidence substantiates to what extent noncompliance with distinct aspects of the dialysis regimen predicts post-transplant noncompliance with the immunosuppressive therapy. More specifically, the few available studies are characterized by a lack of a prospective design and also do not include a valid assessment for noncompliance with the different aspects of the dialysis regimen nor noncompliance with the immunosuppressive regimen, respectively. Most studies also do not state an operational definition of noncompliance or use a composite definition of noncompliance that does not allow understanding of the impact of noncompliance with the distinct aspects of the dialysis regimen on subsequent noncompliance with the post-transplant immunosuppressive therapy. Given these methodological shortcomings, it is not surprising that the few available studies show contradictory results.

Using a retrospective design and chart audit, noncompliance during dialysis and post-transplant noncompliance during a 3 year time period were assessed in 126 adult renal transplant patients [12]. Overall prevalence of pretransplant dialysis noncompliance was 18.3%. Overall prevalence of post-transplant noncompliance was 56%, a rather unexpected high rate admittedly. The rate of 83% documented post-transplant noncompliance in patients who were deemed noncompliant pretransplant contrasts with the 40% post-transplant noncompliance in patients being viewed as compliant pretransplant. In view of the relationship between pretransplant noncompliance and post-transplant outcome, this study found no significant association between pretransplant noncompliance and the rate of post-transplant acute rejection episodes. Yet, graft loss occurred in 43.5% of the patients considered noncompliant pretransplant compared to a rate of 12.6% graft loss in patients deemed compliant pretransplant ($p < 0.01$). Yet, post-transplant compliance is not guaranteed if patients have been compliant during dialysis. Didlake *et al.* [13], as well as Rodin *et al.* [14], reported that patients who were compliant with the dialysis regimen became subsequently non-compliant with the transplant regimen.

Although previous noncompliance is regarded as an important determinant for future noncompliance [11], some caution is indicated in applying this principle blindly in patients with end stage renal disease awaiting transplantation in the absence of reliable empirical evidence. Indeed, the underlying dynamics leading to noncompliance with the distinct aspects of the dialysis regimen can be diverse and quite different from the underlying dynamics resulting in noncompliance with the post-transplant immunosuppressive regimen. For instance, the demands of strict adherence with dietary guidelines and fluid restrictions as part of a dialysis regimen can be particularly burdensome and negatively impact patient's quality of life. Although side effects of the immunosuppressive regimen may also be stressful to patients, the impact of taking immunosuppressive drugs may be perceived as less burdensome and easier to handle in daily life compared to compliance with the various aspects of the dialysis regimen. This might result in satisfactory compliance post-transplant despite noncompliance during dialysis. Vice versa, other dynamics may play a role in patients being perfectly compliant during dialysis who then become noncompliant post-transplant. Moreover, some clinicians perceive that pre-emptive transplantation excluding patients from the dialysis experience with all conditions attached, might be a negative factor in guaranteeing compliance post-transplant. No empirical data are available that do substantiate this perception. Also no evidence is available that addresses differences between modes of dialysis, pre-emptive transplantation and subsequent degree of post-transplant noncompliance with the immunosuppressive regimen.

This lack of evidence does not imply, however, that careful consideration of behavioral aspects of the therapeutic regimen of patients with end-stage renal disease is not indicated. Addressing behavioral issues during dialysis provides a good basis to indicate the importance of patient's adequate self-management during dialysis and to prepare the patient for the responsibilities of the post-transplant therapeutic regimen. Compliance contracts were for instance distributed to poor dialysis compliers by Delone *et al.* [15] and were used as a prerequisite to be placed on the transplant waiting list. Yet, this study did not assess the effectiveness of these contracts.

It is obvious that methodologically sound research is needed to unravel the relationship of noncompliance with the distinct aspects of the dialysis regimen and different treatment modalities for end stage renal disease (*e.g.* hemodialysis, peritoneal dialysis, pre-emptive transplantation) and post-transplant noncompliance with immunosuppressive regimen. Further research efforts should also be devoted in unraveling the underlying dynamics of noncompliance during dialysis and after transplantation. A qualitative approach seems valuable in this regard.

Post-transplant noncompliance as a predictor for subsequent noncompliance and clinical outcome

One-year survival after renal transplantation (RTX) has significantly improved during the last two decades due to more efficacious immunosuppressive drugs. Long-term successful outcome, however, remains jeopardized by acute rejection, chronic rejection and the side effects of the immunosuppressive medication. Noncompliance with the post-transplant regimen, and especially noncompliance with the immunosuppressive drugs, has been recognized as a major risk factor for negative clinical outcome, such as late acute rejection and graft loss. The prevalence of subclinical noncompliance, which refers to patients showing noncompliant behavior, but who do not yet experience a negative clinical event, is substantial, with 20% (range 15-53%) of adult kidney transplant recipients not taking their immunosuppressive drugs as prescribed [13, 16-27]. This rate is even higher in the pediatric renal transplant population, especially in adolescents who show a rate of noncompliance with immunosuppressive drugs up to 64% [28-31].

Depending on case finding and measurement methods used, medication noncompliance is the cause of approximately 20% (range 4.1% to 64%) of late graft failures in adult renal transplant recipients. Of late acute rejection episodes, 34% to 100% have been linked to noncompliance [13, 16-17, 25-27, 32-39]. In the pediatric population, up to 71% of noncompliant patients experienced an acute rejection episode [29] and 6% to 26% of all graft losses have been associated with noncompliance in this patient group [29, 40].

In addition to the negative effects on clinical outcome, limited evidence furthermore shows that noncompliance is associated with higher health care costs [41, 42], yet methodological weaknesses preclude firm conclusions about the exact costs that are associated with noncompliance with the immunosuppressive regimen after renal transplantation.

To our knowledge, only two studies are performed so far assessing the impact of post-transplant noncompliance prospectively on clinical outcome. One study followed patients prospectively from immediately post-transplant up to 5 years after transplantation [43]. Another study focused on patients who were more than one year post-transplant (in process from our research group).

Nevins et al. [43] used electronic event monitoring to substantiate the natural history of azathioprine compliance in a group of 180 renal transplant patients from immediately post-transplant up to 5 years. They determined the impact of early post-transplant compliance on clinical outcome. A low compliance rated during the first 6 months post-transplant was related in a dose-response fashion with acute rejections (p = 0.006) and allograft loss (p = 0.002). Moreover, the adjusted odds for experiencing late acute rejection was 13.9 times higher for patients with declining compliance in the first 90 days post-transplant (95% CI: 2.9-68; p = 0.0011) and the adjusted odds of graft loss was 4.3 times higher (95% CI: 1.1-16; p = 0.0321). These results demonstrate the predictive value of early noncompliance post-transplant for subsequent poor clinical outcome. Moreover, it could be hypothesized that compliance with the immunosuppressive regimen immediately post-transplant is a better predictor for future compliance and clinical outcome than compliance with the various aspects of the dialysis regimen.

Our research group assessed noncompliance with the immunosuppressive regimen in renal transplant patients more than 1 year post-transplant. More specifically, noncompliance with the immunosuppressive regimen was assessed using self-report in 148 patients. Patients were categorized as noncompliers if they stated that they had not taken their immunosuppressive medications correctly during the previous year. The prevalence of medication noncompliance was 22.3% [17]. Patients were subsequently followed-up during a 5 year time period and clinical events were registered. A decreased rejection-free time was observed in noncompliers (log rank: 4.55, p = 0.03). 21.2% of the noncompliers experienced late acute rejections (LAR) at 5 year follow-up compared to 8% of the compliers. Cox regression analysis controlling for time after transplantation and known risk-factors for poor clinical revealed that noncompliance was an independent determinant of in the occurrence of LAR. These preliminary findings suggest that simple interview techniques revealing noncompliance at one time point during the post-transplant course allow to identify a group of patients at risk for poor outcome.

More longitudinal research in transplant populations is needed to further unravel the predictive relationship between noncompliance and negative clinical outcome. Confirmation of this relationship may provide the basis for interventions targeted on high-risk patients.

Noncompliance with immunosuppressive regimen as a predictor for noncompliance after retransplantation

Since transplant registries provide no clear-cut data on the proportion of patients that are retransplanted after renal allograft loss due to noncompliance, it is difficult to assess outcomes of retransplantation in noncompliant patients compared to compliant patients based on registry data to date. To our knowledge, only one single center study assessed the outcome of retransplantation after renal allograft loss due to noncompliance. More specifically, Troppmann et al. [44] reported on the outcome of retransplantation in 14 renal transplant recipients out of a group of 52 patients who lost their graft due to overt noncompliance. These 14 patients were retransplanted if they fulfilled the following four criteria: (1) patient recognition of role of noncompliance in graft failure; (2) current compliance with dialysis regimen; (3) concurrence of all transplant team members that patient was ready for retransplantation; and (4) patient statement to work hard to be compliant and maintain the graft. Eighty-six percent of the patients were compliant after transplantation. Two graft losses occurred, yet noncompliance was not an etiological factor in these events. An overall 1 and 5 year graft and patient survival of 94% and 75%, and of 100% and 100%, respectively was reported.

Retransplantation as a possible therapeutic option for patients who lost their graft due to noncompliance is a subject of intense debate in the realm of distributive justice in times of organ shortage. Some authors state that since noncompliance can be seen as a failure to assume individual responsibility for maintaining health, therefore a noncompliant patient should not be retransplanted [45, 46]. On the other hand, other authors argue that noncompliance can be seen as a disease that can be treated by intervention and that patient would classify for retransplantation after remediation of noncompliance [44].

Compliance interventions

Despite the major progress that has been made in transplant technology, the behavioral pitfall of noncompliance with immunosuppressive therapy remains a major challenge. Overcoming noncompliance provides a clear opportunity to enhance graft survival and to optimize outcomes in renal transplant recipients. Yet, there have been very few intervention studies that test the effectiveness of compliance interventions in transplant populations [15, 29, 31, 47-50]. Moreover, most intervention studies focus on the pediatric transplant population and have been hampered by methodological shortcomings. Thus, though the field of transplantation may start to better understand the genesis of noncompliance, it knows little about how to improve compliance and thus prevent or counter the subsequent occurrence of negative clinical events such as acute rejection or graft loss. Intervention studies to date have focused on isolated educational or social support interventions to enhance compliance, yet with limited success [29, 31, 47-50]. Importantly, there have been no studies of comprehensive, theory-based intervention programs to enhance compliance with immunosuppressive medication. Yet, empirical evidence from other chronic patient populations underscores the feasibility and effectiveness of compliance interventions for specific medication regimens [51-54]. Specifically, interventions should aim at combining educational, behavioral and social support interventions. This should be done using both the available evidence about modifiable determinants of noncompliance and the limited evidence from randomized clinical trials to enhance medication compliance in chronic patient populations [53, 54]. Empirical evidence shows that the use of electronic event monitoring as a combined monitoring and intervention tool is effective in improving compliance in hypertensive and psychiatric patients [55, 56].

Conclusions

Noncompliance is an important clinical risk factor during the illness course of patients with end stage renal disease. There is a definite need for further research to substantiate the contribution of noncompliance on outcome during the different phases of end-stage renal disease. Moreover, an urgent need is identified to test the effectiveness of compliance interventions to enhance long-term successful outcome after transplantation.

References

1. Schneider MS, *et al.* Fluid noncompliance and symptomatology in end-stage renal disease: cognitive and emotional variables. *Health Psychol* 1991; 10: 209-15.
2. Bame SI, *et al.* Variation in hemodialysis patient compliance according to demographic characteristics. *Soc Sci Med* 1993; 37: 1035-43.
3. Christensen AJ, *et al.* Coping with treatment related stress: effects on patient adherence in hemodialysis. *J Consult Clin Psychol* 1995; 63: 454-9.
4. Leggat JE, *et al.* Non-compliance in hemodialysis: predictors and survival analysis. *Am J Kidney Dis* 1998; 32: 139-45.
5. Brown J, *et al.* Factors influencing compliance with dietary restrictions in dialysis patients. *Psychosom Res* 1988; 32: 191-6.
6. Tracy HM, *et al.* Noncompliance in hemodialysis patients as measured with MBHI. *Psychol Health* 1987; 1: 411-23.
7. Briggs JD. Patient selection for renal transplantation. *Nephrol Dial Transplant* 1995; 10 (Suppl. 1): 10-3.
8. Ramos EL *et al.* The evaluation of candidates for renal transplantation. *Transplantation* 1994; 57: 490-7.
9. Hathaway DK, *et al.* Patient compliance in transplantation: a report of the perceptions of transplant clinicians. *Transplant Proc* 1999; 31 (Suppl. 4A): 10S-3.
10. Thamer M, *et al.* US nephrologists' attitudes towards renal transplantation: results from a national survey. *Transplantation* 2001; 71: 281-8.
11. Dunbar-Jacob J. Predictors of patient adherence. Patient characteristics. In: Shumaker SA, Schron EB, Ockene JK, eds. *The handbook of health behavior change.* Springer, New York, 1990: 348-60.
12. Douglas S, *et al.* Relationship between pre-transplant noncompliance and post-transplant outcomes in renal transplant recipients. *J Transplant Coordin* 1996; 6: 53-8.

13. Didlake RH, et al. Patient noncompliance: a major cause of late graft failure in Cyclosporine-treated renal transplants. *Transplant Proc* 1988; 10 (Suppl. 3): 63-9.
14. Rodin G, et al. Kidney transplantation. In: Craven J, Rodin GM, eds. *Psychiatric aspects of organ transplantation.* Oxford: Oxford University Press, 1992: 145.
15. Delone P, et al. Non-compliance in renal transplant recipients: methods for recognition and intervention. *Transplant Proc* 1989; 21: 3982-4.
16. Kiley DJ, et al. A study of treatment compliance following kidney transplantation. *Transplantation* 1993; 55: 51-6.
17. De Geest S, et al. Incidence, determinants, and consequences of subclinical noncompliance with immunosuppressive therapy in renal transplant recipients. *Transplantation* 1995; 59: 340-7.
18. Greenstein S, et al. Odds probabilities of noncompliance in patients with a functioning renal transplant: a multicenter study. *Transplant Proc* 1999; 31: 280-1.
19. Greenstein S, et al. Compliance and noncompliance in patients with a functioning renal transplant: a multicenter study. *Transplantation* 1998; 27: 1718-26.
20. Hilbrands LB, et al. Medication compliance after renal transplantation. *Transplantation* 1995; 60: 914-20.
21. Rovelli M, et al. Noncompliance in organ transplant recipients. *Transplant Proc* 1989; 21: 833-4.
22. Schweizer RT, et al. Noncompliance in organ transplant recipients. *Transplantation* 1990; 49: 374-7.
23. Siegal BR. Postrenal transplant compliance: report of 519 responses to a self-report questionnaire. *Transplantation Proc* 1993; 25: 2502.
24. Swanson AM, et al. Noncompliance in organ transplant recipients. *Pharmacotherapy* 1991; 11: 173S-4.
25. Dunn J, et al. Causes of graft loss beyond two years in the cyclosporine era. *Transplantation* 1990; 49: 349-53.
26. Garcia V, et al. Patient noncompliance as a major cause of kidney graft failure. XVI International Congress of the Transplantation Society, Barcelona, 1996, Abstract 85.
27. Hong JH, et al. Causes of late renal allograft failure in the ciclosporin era. *Nephron* 1992; 62: 272-9.
28. Foulkes LM, et al. Social support, family variables, and compliance in renal transplant children. *Pediatr Nephrol* 1993; 7: 185-8.
29. Ettenger RB, et al. Improved cadaveric renal transplant outcome in children. *Pediatr Nephrol* 1991; 5: 137-42.
30. Blowley DL, et al. Compliance with cyclosporine in adolescent renal transplant recipients. *Pediatr Nephrol* 1997; 11: 547-51.
31. Beck DE, et al. Evaluation of an educational program on compliance with medication regimens in pediatric patients with renal transplants. *J Pediatr* 1980; 96: 1094-1097.
32. Bittar AE, et al. Patient noncompliance as a cause of late kidney graft failure. *Transplant Proceed* 1992; 24: 2710-21.
33. Gaston RS, et al. Late renal allograft loss: noncompliance masquerading as chronic rejection. *Transplant Proceed* 1999; 31 (Suppl. 4A): 21S-3.
34. Peeters J, et al. Chronic renal allograft failure: clinical overview. The Leuven Collaborative Group for Transplantation. *Kidney Int* 1995; 52 (Suppl.): S97-101.
35. Shoskes DA, et al. Patient death or renal allograft loss within 3 years of transplantation in a county hospital: importance of poor initial graft function. *Clin Transplant* 1997; 11: 618-22.
36. Bregmann L, et al. Late graft loss in cadaveric renal transplantation. *Transplant Proceed* 1992; 24: 2718-9.
37. Burke JF, et al. Long-term efficacy and safety of cyclosporine in renal transplant recipients. *N Engl J Med* 1994; 331: 358-63.
38. Dunn J, et al. Long-term benefit and risks of cyclosporine therapy. In: Paul LC et al., eds. *Organ transplantation. Long-term results.* New York: Marcel Dekker, 1992: 85-98.
39. Isaacs RB, et al. Noncompliance in living-related donor renal transplantation: the UNOS experience. *Transplant Proceed* 1999; 31 (Suppl. 4A): 19S-20.
40. Gagnadoux MF, et al. Non-immunological risk factors in pediatric renal transplantation. *Pediatr Nephrol* 1993; 7: 89-95.
41. Swanson M, et al. Economic impact of noncompliance in kidney transplant recipients. *Transplant Proceed* 1992; 24: 2722.
42. Brickman AL, et al. Noncompliance in end-stage renal disease: a threat to quality of care and cost containment. *J Clin Psychol Med Settings* 1996; 3: 399-412.
43. Nevins TE, et al. Medication compliance after transplantation. *Clin Transplant* 2001; in press.

44. Troppmann C, *et al.* Retransplantation after renal allograft loss due to noncompliance. Indications, outcome, and ethical concerns. *Transplantation* 1995; 59: 467-71.
45. Bromberg JS, *et al.* Renal transplantation in a noncompliant patient. *N Engl J Med* 1994; 330: 371.
46. Evans RW. A cost-outcome analysis of retransplantation: the need of accountability. *Transplantation Rev* 1993; 7: 163.
47. Fennell RS, *et al.* Family-based program to promote medication compliance in renal transplant children. *Transplant Proceed* 1994; 26: 102-3.
48. Steinberg TG, *et al.* An evaluation of the effectiveness of a videotape for discharge teaching of organ transplant recipients. *J Transplant Coordin* 1996; 6: 59-63.
49. Goldstein NL, *et al.* Comparison of two teaching strategies: adherence to a home monitoring program. *Clin Nursing Res* 1996; 5: 150-66.
50. Traiger GL, *et al.* A self-medication administration program for transplant recipients. *Crit Care Nurse* 1997; 17: 71-9.
51. Dunbar-Jacob J, *et al.* Clinical assessment and management of adherence to medical regimens. In: Nicassio PM, Smith TW, eds. *Managing chronic illness: abiopsychosocial perspective.* Washington DC: American Psychological Association, 1995.
52. Haynes RB, *et al.* Systematic review of randomized trials of interventions to assist patients to follow prescriptions for medications. *Lancet* 1996; 348: 383-6.
53. Haynes RB, *et al.* Interventions for helping patients to follow prescriptions for medications (Cochrane Review). In: The Cochrane Library, Issue 2, 2000. Oxford: Update Software.
54. Roter DL, *et al.* Effectiveness of interventions to improve patient compliance: a meta-analysis. *Med Care* 1998; 36: 1138-61.
55. Cramer JA, *et al.* Enhancing medication compliance with serious mental illness. *J Nervous Mental Dis* 1999; 187: 52-4.
56. Burnier M, *et al.* Electronic compliance monitoring in resistant hypertension: the basis for rational therapeutic decisions. *J Hypertens* 2001; 19: 335-41.

Predicting the natural course of nephrotic syndrome in children. An integrate clinical and molecular approach

Gian Marco Ghiggeri, Francesco Perfumo
Nephrology Unit, Giannina Gaslini Children Hospital, Genoa, Italy

The term nephrotic syndrome (NS) identifies a clinical condition characterized by the classical triad of proteinuria, diffuse edema due to hyponchia, and dislipidemia, that in children is mostly referred to the so-called minimal change (MCD) – focal sclerosis (FSGS) complex. This is a potentially heterogeneous group of diseases which has not been definitely characterized yet. However, it is possible to differentiate separate clinical entities on the basis of the outcome that is strictly dependent on the sensitivity to therapeutical approaches and is probably related to different pathogenetic mechanisms.

In the past a classification based on drug response and on hystological elements has been privileged; nowadays, following some improvements on the knowledge of the pathogenetic mechanisms, it seems possible that further elements on molecular aspects of podocyte components and on biochemistry of plasma factors for glomerular permeability could improve our classificatory effort. This review will summarize how these different elements may contribute to our conceptual and practical approach to NS in children focusing on the following point: 1) drug response and pathology; 2) molecular mechanisms of proteinuria linked to proteins of the podocyte; 3) humoral factors with permeability activity and 4) associations with pro-sclerotic substances.

Drug response and pathology, two complementary aspects of NS

Drug response remains the basic criterion for a proper classification of NS in children, with evident therapeutical and prognostic consequences. Steroid responsiveness makes the difference on prognosis. In the late 70's, multicentric studies have defined the best conditions for steroids, including doses and times of the assumption, and, with minor changes, this remains the usual therapeutical approach [1, 2].

Between the two extreme responses, *i.e.* prompt remission- absolute resistance, there are forms that respond to steroids but present frequent relapses and forms which are strictly dependent to steroids and need a continuous drug support. A simplified classification of NS in children should consider the following three categories: a) steroid responsiveness with sustained remission or unfrequent relapses; b) steroids and cyclosporin resistance; c) steroid resistance or strict dependence, with responsiveness to cyclosporin. Group "a" has always a good outcome in terms of persistence of proteinuria and progression of the renal disease; group "b" almost invariably shows an outcome to renal failure. Prognosis in group "c" is strictly dependent to the sensitivity of the host to respond to low levels of cyclosporin and to the possibility to follow long term regimen with the drug, that means absence of tubulo-interstitial fibrosis after 5 or more years of therapy.

Glucocorticoid receptors (GCr) may be a determinant of the differential response to the steroids. Indeed, cell response is influenced by both levels and structure of GCr, their affinity for ligands and transcriptional properties [3]. We also know that GCr expression varies in different tissues and no specific study has so far addressed the problem in kidneys of nephrotic children. However, the density of GCr in mononuclear cells was reported to reflect the *"in vivo"* effects of steroids in healthy humans and in various diseases, including lupus nephritis [4]. The data so far available on NS are conflictual; the most recent and probably technically advanced study [5] demonstrates that the density of GCr is similar in children with different types of NS, including the steroid resistant type, thus suggesting no predictive value in steroid response and hence in long term outcome.

Renal pathology does not represent *per se* an efficient prognostic criterion. It varies from minimal lesions only visible with electron microscopy, to mesangial proliferation with IgM deposits and to glomerulosclerosis. A major bias for the classification of NS based on pathology is sampling, since glomerulosclerotic lesions, even in severe cases, may involve less than 5% of all glomeruli and any hystological sample containing less than 10 glomeruli could not be representative of the whole population. In general, focal glomerulosclerosis occurs in patients with steroid resistance and "vice versa" minimal changes are typical of easy and sustained steroid responsiveness but cases with FSGS and quiescent disease after steroids are not infrequent. However, histological patterns of groups "b" and "c" may overlap in patients who respond to cyclosporin and, in these cases, it is difficult to define a natural history on prognostic bases. Moreover, the typical lesion of FSGS may be absent, initially, on biopsy of children with NS who are resistant to steroids and may reflect the progressive nature of the disease process. In a series of 49 patients who received more than one renal biopsy, Ahmad and Tejani [6] found that the initial minimal change lesions evolved to IgM nephropathy in 7 and to FSGS in 14 cases. Therefore, the renal biopsy may facilitate diagnosis when definite lesions are present; but in the case of normal histology the interpretation is problematic.

In summary, drug response to steroids represents a basic point to attempt a reasonable prognosis in NS and renal pathology is an additional element that may confirm and compendiate the original conclusion, but problems in sampling and the possibility of evolving lesions depending on time of the procedure reduce its overall value in clinical setting. Responsiveness to cyclosporin has changed the natural course of NS in patients with corticodependence and in some cases with corticoresistance, but its impact on the long term prognosis of the disease has to be defined yet.

Podocyte protein composition, the new mechanism for proteinuria and possible prediction

The podocyte and the slit diaphragm have now been recognized as the effective site with repulsive functions against proteins in glomeruli [7-9]. Functional and molecular characterization of single components of podocytes would represent the new frontier in the attempt to define criteria for guessing the natural course of NS. This means that an early identification of molecular defects in proteins that govern the permeability functions or the definition of regulatory mechanisms mediated by immunologic factors or by drugs should strengthen our prognostic approach to the disease.

Seminal work on congenital nephrotic syndrome of the Finnish type, done by the Finnish group of Tryggvason, has first identified nephrin as the major constituent of the so-called interpodocyte-zipper structure for repulsion [8]. Successive studies by Kaplan and Pollack [10] and by Boute and Antignac [11] identified other podocyte proteins which play a pivotal role in the maintenance of glomerular impermeability. The up-to-date list includes podocin and α-actinin 4, whose mutations are responsible for familiar forms of NS with autosomal recessive and dominant inheritance respectively, and CD2AP [12] that is responsible for proteinuria in rats.

We now also know that homozygous and heterozygous mutations of podocin are frequent in children with sporadic NS and that the NPHS2 gene is rich in polymorphisms and single nucleotide polymorphisms (SNPs) that may have functional consequences [13]. *Table I* shows the major mutations of podocin found in an Italian population with sporadic NS that had been classified as having FSGS before the molecular analysis on NPHS2 was available.

All patients with homozygous mutations of podocin presented drug unresponsiveness and progression to end stage renal failure. Heterozygous mutations and polymorphisms may determine variability in regulation of podocin levels in podocyte and may represent an important prognostic factor in NS. Finally, patients with early onset NS with concomitant mutations in heterozygosity of nephrin and podocin have been reported; therefore, children bearing a heterozygous mutation of podocin should also be tested for mutations in nephrin. Synaptopodin is another component of the podocyte cytoskeleton that may bring about prognostic potential. It is a proline-rich protein intimately associated with the actin filaments that are believed to modulate the shape and mobility of foot-processes. A decrease or loss of synaptopodin had been observed in FSGS, collapsing FSGS and in HIV-associated nephropathy. Synaptopodin expression is also decreased in FSGS compared to minimal changes [14]. Thus, it appears that synaptopodin expression is not a part of a primary process but it is rather a secondary phenomenon that reflects the magnitude of the damage. In this view, synaptopodin may be potentially useful as a marker to evaluate the cellular alteration in podocytes and to predict the steroid response of NS.

Minor molecular conditions responsible for NS resistant to steroids are related to abnormalities of mitochrondrial DNA [16] and to WT1 [17], but these are very rare occurrences that should be suspected in patients with a family history and involvement of unrelated tissues such as muscles or gonads.

Recurrence of the Disease in the Renal Graft
Cochat P, ed.
© John Libbey Eurotext, Paris, 2001

Podocyte injury underlies progression of chronic renal disease. Evidence from experimental models

Wilhelm Kriz
Institut für Anatomie und Zellbiologie, Universität Heidelberg, Germany

Progression of glomerular diseases to end-stage renal failure is underlain by the progressive loss of viable nephrons. To understand this process, two phases of nephron loss have to be distinguished. First, a phase in which the mechanisms of nephron loss are disease-specific (glomerulonephritis, diabetes). This phase lasts as long as the loss of nephrons does not necessitate overload work by the remaining nephrons. The second one, the progressive phase, begins as soon as the compensatory work of the remaining nephrons, during or after a specific disease, results in an overload that *per se* initiates or at least contributes to the degeneration of further nephrons.

The general mechanisms in the second phase (which may become additive if the primary disease is still flourishing) appear to be essentially based on an overload function of the glomerulus. Glomerular hypertrophy, glomerular hypertension and hyperfiltration appear to be the major factors accounting for the progressive loss of nephrons. These factors are frequently relevant also to nephron degeneration in the transplanted kidney.

There are basically two theories as to the mechanisms underlying nephron loss in the second phase: (i) protein leakage associated with glomerular malfunction due to overload leads to long term lasting protein reabsorbtion by proximale tubules, which become injured. They start to secrete mediators, that initiate interstitial proliferation and matrix deposition leading to progressive renal fibrosis. Thus, progression of the disease is sustained by a selfperpetuating process of the tubulointerstitium; (ii) glomerular malfunction due to overload initiates a damaging process in the glomerulus itself, thus also in the second phase the degeneration of the glomerulus is the essential event, degeneration of the tubule is secondary.

The role of the tubulo interstitium in progressive nephron loss

The hypothesis is widely favored that local tubulo-interstitial mechanisms, notably interstitial proliferation and matrix deposition, are the dominating processes leading to progressive renal scarring followed by the loss of further nephrons. Thus, even if initiated by a glomerular injury due to glomerular overload function, it is finally a tubulo-interstitial process which accounts for the degeneration of the affected nephrons [1-6]. The most frequently discussed concept as to how the injury which originates in the glomerulus spreads to the tubulo-interstitium suggests that glomerular protein leakage represents the decisive link between glomerular and tubulo-interstitial injury [1-3, 7]. Glomeruli with glomerular hypertension and hyperfiltration allow continuous leakage of plasma proteins into the tubular urine leading to continuous protein reabsorption by the proximal tubules. In response, the tubules secrete mediators (such as monocyte chemokine protein type I, platelet derived growth factor, osteopontin, endothelin and others) towards the interstitium, giving rise to interstitial proliferation and matrix deposition. These processes – in addition to being responsible for the final destruction of the already affected nephron – initiate destructive mechanisms in neighboring nephrons now starting at the tubule [1, 2, 6, 7].

The evidence for such a mechanism is weak. No question, persistent protein leakage through the glomerular filter leads to persistent protein reabsorption and degradation by the corresponding proximal tubule. It may well be that this persistent protein reabsorption is a damaging factor to the affected proximal tubule. However – and this is quite clear from our many studies that include experimental models as well as human cases of FSGS [8, 9] –, interstitial proliferation, as it locally occurs in the surroundings of injured tubules and glomeruli, even in the vicinity of tubules with excessive protein reabsorption, does not appear to exert damaging effects onto neighboring healthy tubules. To state it otherwise: intact tubules encountered amidst groups of injured tubular profiles with protein reabsorption and surrounding fibrosis do not appear to become affected by the tubulo-interstitial process in their immediate vicinity. A major argument against the nephron-to-nephron transfer of the disease at the level of the tubulo-interstitium is represented by the fact that a sequence of damaging events which might account for the encroachment of a focal tubular injury, mediated by interstitial proliferation or any other mechanism, onto a neighboring nephron, tubule or glomerulus, has never been published and has not become obvious to us in our studies.

Progressive podocyte loss underlies the entry of nephrons into the pathway to degeneration

There are many and convincing results from studies in humans and animals documenting a major influence of glomerular protein leakage on progression, more precisely, documenting a remarkable deceleration of progression when protein leakage is reduced [7, 10-14]. If, as our studies suggest, there is no nephron to nephron transfer of the disease at the level of the tubulo-interstitium, the only other site where sustained protein leakage might have damaging effects to a given nephron is the glomerulus itself.

Within a list of possible factors damaging a podocyte under the conditions of FSGS development, an exuberant lysosomal uptake of proteins passing through a nearby damaged filter A [15, 16] has ranged at a prominent position. Since the classic experimental study by Farquhar and Palade in 1961 [17], podocytes densely filled with absorption granules have been encountered in many experimental glomerular diseases including all models of FSGS [16, 18-22] and are well known in the pathology of human cases. Evidence for the rupture of lysosomal elements, spillage of lysosomal enzymes and subsequent dissolution of such podocytes have also been presented previously [16]. Moreover, as seen in our studies and in those from others [17, 21] podocytes filled with lysosomal elements consistently display additional injuries, such as foot process effacement and formation of pseudocysts.

Based on these observations and the lack of evidence that local interstitial proliferation in the context of nephron degeneration in FSGS is damaging to healthy nephrons, we propose that persistent protein leakage through an injured glomerular filter may exert damaging effects on podocytes by seducing them to excessive endocytotic protein uptake and lysosomal digestion, thereby exposing them to the danger of spillage of lysosomal enzymes out of an excessively developed lysosomal system into the cytoplasm, as has been suggested for the proximal tubule [2].

Thus, this proposal includes a self-perpetuating mechanism of renal destruction fully compatible with the self-perpetuating model of renal destruction advanced by Brenner et al. [23]. Glomerular hypertension results in a lasting pressure challenge to podocytes leading to protein leakage, leading to further podocyte damage. Thus, protein leakage probably is a decisive mediator between increases in glomerular pressure and podocyte injury.

Moreover, recent work has supported the long-standing observations that in experimental models, as well as in human cases of proteinuric diseases, ACE inhibitors have renoprotective properties beyond systemic blood pressure reduction [24-29]. There is increasing evidence that these additional beneficial effects of ACE inhibitors stem from the improvement of the glomerular filter, thus lowering the protein leakage through the filter. The site and the mechanism, by which these effects are brought about, are a matter of debate. First, there is evidence that it is indeed the blockage of ANGII and not of bradykinin that accounts for the positive effects [24, 30]. Moreover, there is increasing evidence that these positive effects result from preservation of podocyte function. In PHN [26] ACE inhibitors prevented structural changes of podocytes (decrease in filtration slit frequency). Moreover, aging male MWF rats develop spontaneous proteinuria, which is associated with cellular changes in podocytes such as the redistribution of ZO-1 from its usual location at the slit membrane into the cytoplasm [27]. This redistribution as well as proteinuria and further sclerosis development were hindered by treatment with ACE inhibitors. In addition, beneficial effects of ACE inhibitors were noted in adriamycin nephropathy, where they prevent the loss of heparan sulfate proteoglycans from the GBM [30]. Taken together, these observations suggest that the renoprotective effects of ACE inhibitors are mediated at the podocyte.

The pathway of nephron degeneration starting from podocyte injury

So far we have discussed that continuous podocyte injury is the most probable cause of progressive nephron loss in end stage renal failure. We have not discussed how podocyte injury leads to the degeneration of the entire nephron.

There are at least two basically different pathways how podocyte injury may lead to nephron loss – one characteristic for inflammatory glomerular diseases, the other characteristic for degenerative glomerular diseases. Formation of glomerular crescents and subsequence strangulation of the affected glomerulus represent the inflammatory pathway [31]. Characteristic for the overload phase in progressive renal disease is the de-

and 80% of the children attended a normal school. Those children who had neurological problems belonged to the very first patients treated at our institution, and they had thrombotic complications prior to the introduction of routine anticoagulation from the first weeks of life [14]. When analyzing the causes of graft loss it was obvious that the main problem in NPHS1 patients was recurrence of proteinuria in the new kidney, sometimes leading to graft loss.

Post-transplant proteinuria in NPHS1 patients

In 1989 Sigström et al. reported recurrence of proteinuria in a child with CNF [14], leading to loss of the graft and proteinuria has recurred in two subsequent grafts in this child (personal communication). In 1993, when 29 renal transplantations had been performed in CNF patients at our institution, we reported recurrence of proteinuria in seven grafts [15]. Many of the patients had had a recent CMV infection. Four episodes responded to cyclophosphamide therapy, when this was instituted instead of azathioprine in their triple immunosuppression, but three grafts were lost.

Isolation of the NPHS1 gene and localization of nephrin to the slit diaphragm made further characterization of the pathogenesis of proteinuria after renal transplantation in NPHS1 patients possible. Patrakka investigated all our 45 NPHS1 patients receiving 51 kidney transplants between 1986 and 2000 [16]. In these patients, 15 episodes of recurrent proteinuria occurred in 13 grafts (25%). All nine patients with recurrence were homozygotes for the Fin-major mutation. Rescue therapy with cyclophosphamide was successful in 7 episodes of recurrent proteinuria (47%), but six kidneys were lost because of this process. Thus, graft survival in Fin-major homozygotes has been only 72% and nephrosis has recurred in 37% of their grafts [16]. In contrast, graft survival has thus far been 100% in the 16 NPHS1 patients with other mutations and transplanted at our institution.

In Alport's syndrome, caused by mutations in the gene(s) coding for type IV collagen about 10% of the patients develop *de novo* anti-GBM disease because of an immune response against the previously unseen collagen epitopes in the kidney graft [17]. Thus, we postulated that in the Fin-major homozygotes, where no nephrin is expressed in the native kidney, an immune response against nephrin in the graft may develop in some patients. Fetuses with the Fin-major genotype do not encounter nephrin during normal maturation of their immunological system, and do not develop tolerance to nephrin. When nephrin is exposed in the kidney graft after transplantation, immunization against this "novel" antigen may occur.

In accordance with this theory Patrakka was able to find anti-nephrin antibodies in four of the nine patients with recurrence, with the ELISA-method [16]. Three children had two episodes and the latter occurred soon (5-31 days) after retransplantation in contrast to the first episodes, after their first renal transplantation, which mostly occurred 6 to 48 months after transplantation. This suggests that preformed antibodies might play a pathogenic role. Anti-nephrin antibodies could not be demonstrated in five patients with recurrent proteinuria, using the extracellular part of the nephrin molecule as antigen in the assay. However, in four of these patients, antibodies against fetal glomerulus could be demonstrated by immunofluorescence. It has also been shown in rats that after injection of antibody 5-1-6, directed against the extracellular domain of rat nephrin, proteinuria develops within days [18, 19]. However, immunoglobulin or complement deposits could not be demonstrated in the proteinuric grafts of our patients. It is thus possible that the amount of the antibodies involved may be small and, perhaps, the antibodies are lost in the urine. Also, regulatory T-cells might control the immune responsiveness to nephrin and this might explain why recurrence of NS occurs in only some patients with the Fin-major/Fin-major genotype.

Histologically the glomeruli looked quite normal at light microscopy in biopsies taken within a few days after the start of proteinuria [15]. On electron microscopy, effacement of the podocyte foot processes was evident and the frequency of slit pores, devoid of filamentous image of the slit diaphragm was clearly increased. In addition, junctions with ladder-like structures [16] were occasionally observed between the podocytes. These findings suggest that disruption of the slit diaphragm takes place, and possibly leads to foot process fusion, and proteinuria.

Treatment of post-transplant proteinuria?

If cyclophosphamide was instituted in addition to the normal methylprednisolone and cyclosporine medication early after recurrence, remission could be achieved in about 50% of the patients [15, 16]. Most of these patients remained in remission, but some relapsed, and some of these relapses responded to a new course of cyclophosphamide. Treatment of patients with preformed antibodies against nephrin and recurrence of nephrosis in subsequent transplantations constitute a difficult problem. In one patient we instituted methylprednisolone, cyclosporine and cyclophosphamide and performed plasmapheresis 2-3 times a week for several weeks, in addition to prophylactic gancyclovir to avoid additional CMV infection. Although proteinuria appeared during the first week after retransplantation it slowly decreased and this patient is presently doing all right, with minimal proteinuria (145 mg/day) and slightly reduced renal function (GFR = 63 ml/min/1.73 m^2) two years after his second renal transplantation.

We are currently following the anti-nephrin antibodies in NPHS1 patients with the Fin-major/Fin-major genotype after renal transplantation. However, with the present technique a clear correlation between antibody titer and proteinuria cannot yet be found. In patients with recurrent proteinuria unresponsive to therapy one might consider to use immunoglobuline infusions (IVIG), which have been successfully used to inhibit HLA-specific antibodies in highly sensitized transplant patients [20, 21].

Conclusion

Post-transplant proteinuria in NPHS1 patients seems to occur only in patients who have not encountered nephrin during normal maturation, like patients with the Fin-major/Fin-major genotype. In these patients proteinuria occurs in the graft in about 30%. Formation of anti-nephrin antibodies seems to play a main role in this process, and leads to disruption of the slit diaphragm, and proteinuria. Early cyclophosphamide therapy, sometimes combined with plasmapheresis and possibly IVIG infusions often reverses proteinuria.

lity of primary SRNS and skip directly to the secondary pathologic effects resulting from a common pathway of progressive renal injury.

Thus we are left with the difficult task of studying post-transplant recurrent SRNS in the complex setting of patient-based research, with inherent disadvantages including imperfect controls and multiple confounding variables. Given the significant impact of this disease process in the pediatric renal transplant population, the importance and difficulty of this task cannot be understated. While there have been some intriguing advances in our understanding of post-transplant NS, much more has yet to be delineated. However, our current understanding of this disorder can be grouped into genetic, structural, circulating and immunologic factors.

Genetic and structural factors

A familial form of NS has been described relatively recently. Linkage analysis has provided evidence suggesting that a mutation that causes autosomal dominant FSGS is located on human chromosome 19q13 (locus FSGS-1) based on studies in a large family from Oklahoma [16]. Genotyping of family members at markers on chromosome 19q13 narrowed the candidate interval to a 3.5-Mb region flanked by D19S609 and D19S417. In one additional small family from California, the disease segregated with chromosome 19q13.1 marker alleles. Mutations in the gene encoding α-actinin-4 (ACTN4) on chromosome 19q13.1 were then described as the cause of FSGS in three families with an autosomal dominant form of FSGS [17]. ACTN4 is an actin-filament crosslinking protein. Based on actin-binding experiments, it was concluded that these mutations result in altered regulation of the actin cytoskeleton of glomerular podocytes, the epithelial cells that play a key role in the glomerular basement membrane. The clinical manifestations of familial FSGS are extremely variable, ranging from virtual absence of clinical disease to rapid progression to ESRD[18]. To date, there are no reports of recurrent disease following transplantation, distinguishing familial FSGS from primary FSGS.

It has been postulated that patients with inherited or spontaneous mutations may be predisposed to nephrotic syndrome that would manifest as primary SRNS [19]. The observation that recurrence of SRNS following transplantation may be more likely to occur in recipients of kidneys from related donors compared with recipients of cadaveric kidneys [6, 20] supports this hypothesis to some extent. Alternatively, one could hypothesize that mutations associated with familial or congenital nephrotic syndrome result in a structural abnormality localized to some key component of the glomerular basement membrane, based on the absence of recurrence following transplantation of kidneys from either related or unrelated donors. Conversely, primary SRNS clearly appears to be a systemic disorder in that anephric patients often experience recurrence within days of receiving an allograft. It remains likely that all NS represent a group of genetically heterogeneous disorders with similar phenotypes.

Immunohistochemistry analyses of graft tissue obtained from six subjects with post-transplant recurrent SRNS revealed several interesting structural findings, including detached podocytes, loss of podocyte-specific epitopes, increased expression of several cytokeratins, and expression of macrophagic epitopes by numerous cells in Bowman's space and within tubular lumens [21]. These data suggest that podocytes may be dysregulated in some way in SRNS relapsing after transplantation.

Circulating factors

The short median time to recurrence along with the significant beneficial effects of systemic therapy on proteinuria in post-transplant recurrent SRNS strongly suggest that a circulating factor or group of factors is involved in the pathogenesis of SRNS. Both protein A adsorption[22] and plasmapharesis[23, 24] have been used to isolate and study the characteristics of the plasma factor(s) which may mediate proteinuria. *In vivo* assays have shown that the permeability factor(s) rapidly induce proteinuria when injected into rodents [22]. More recently, however, it has been suggested that *in vivo* injection of circulating substances into rodents is not a reliable model for testing plasma fraction activity [25].

An ingenious *in vitro* model involving isolated glomeruli provides a clinically applicable assay of glomerular permeability, termed "$P_{albumin}$" [23, 24]. $P_{albumin}$ is significantly higher in serum from patients with recurrent FSGS compared with serum from patients without recurrence or from normal controls, and plasmapharesis significantly reduces the $P_{albumin}$ in parallel with a decrease in proteinuria [24]. The inhibitory effect of CsA on $P_{albumin}$ is impressive and is associated with increased glomerular cyclic AMP [26, 27]. Another innovative *in vitro* assay has been devised which measures the effect of patients' serum on glomerular volume variation (GVV). The serum GVV is significantly higher in patients with SRNS compared with control groups and other glomerular and non-glomerular diseases, although there is significant variability within the SRNS group. Incubation of rat mesangial cells with circulating factor obtained from patients with post-transplant recurrent SRNS inhibited nitrite accumulation, with a parallel decrease in inducible nitric oxide synthase gene expression and protein levels [28], suggesting that a circulating factor may affect glomerular permselectivity and/or matrix protein synthesis.

The questions remaining regarding circulating factors include: (1) What are the exact molecular and genetic characteristics of the circulating factor(s)? (2) What is/are the cell(s) of origin? (3) Why is it expressed in SRNS/FSGS? (4) What are the target cells, receptors, and intracellular mechanisms involved that result in proteinuria?

Immunologic factors

Several immunologic irregularities and cytokine changes have been reported as potential pathophysiologic mechanisms of post-transplant recurrent SRNS. Treatment of post-transplant recurrence with sequential use of non-protein A anti-Ig affinity columns, followed by protein A immunoadsorption in four subjects with recurrent disease demonstrated comparable effects on proteinuria, and on depletion of plasma factors capable of altering albumin permselectivity in isolated glomeruli [29]. This suggests that immunoglobulins likely are involved in the complex interplay between circulating factors and proteinuria.

Circulating factor isolated, partially identified, and proteinuria induced in normal rats

Bakker *et al.* [2] have described a serum factor, which they have called 100 KF. It is present in normal human, in patients with LN both in remission and in relapse, and also in rat serum. It is secreted by the hepatocyte.

This factor has been infused using a cannula placed in the suprarenal artery. The factor or albumin (BSA as control) were infused using high flow rates (5 to 20 ml/hr). After infusing the factor, they observed an increase in urinary albumin excretion.

The clinical significance of this factor is questionable because the author observed decreased 100 KF levels during relapse as compared with samples from patients in remission. The patients in remission had 100KF levels within the range of values observed in normal controls. It is not clear, then, how a factor at reduced concentrations will cause the effect on proteinuria not seen at higher concentrations. The authors have suggested that the low levels are due to an increase catabolism. However, to this date, there are no data on the factor catabolic rate in LN patients in relapse.

Circulating factor isolated, identified?, proteinuria induced in the experimental animal [3, 4]?

A factor(s) has(ve) been postulated to be present in the circulation of some patients with nephrotic syndrome and FGSG who progress into renal failure. When these patients are transplanted, within a short period of time after transplantation (from hours to a few days), they developed proteinuria. Moreover, when these patients undergo plasmapheresis, proteinuria decreases significantly.

Effect of the circulating factor on urinary protein excretion in the experimental animal

• Columns for inmmunoadsorption of circulating material (protein A or immunoglobulin affinity columns) have been used during plasmapheresis to isolate the factor. After eluting the column, Dantal *et al.* isolated a factor from the molecules retained in the protein A column. When these isolated substances were infused into rats by single injection, an increase in albuminuria was seen.

• Factor isolated from plasma of patients with FSGS. Both Savin and Dantal have isolated, concentrated, and enriched a factor after sequential removal of the cryoproteins, lipoproteins and chylomicrons, IgG, and albumin rich protein fractions of the plasma obtained during plasmapheresis. Both have injected same fraction (70% supernatant fraction) to rats with opposite results. Savin administered the concentrated supernatant intravenously. As control, supernatant from plasma of normal subjects was used. The single injection of the supernatant from same patient to different rats was followed by an increase in total urinary protein excretion. According to the size of the observed SEM, the intratest results (supernatant from same patients tested several times) vary widely. "t" test (instead of nonparametric statistics) was used to analyze the data.

Dantal group injected the same volume of same 70% supernatant fraction *ex vivo*, intraperitoneally, and intravenously. They measured both albumin and total protein. Appropriately, non-parametric statistics were used to analyze the data and no concentrated supernatant was injected more than once. An increase in urinary protein was observed when fraction from FSGS patients was administered, but also when fraction from normal individuals and saline. Borderline changes in urinary protein excretion were seen when fraction from patients with nephrotic syndrome other than FSGS was infused.

Characterization of the circulating factor

Savin has reported to have isolated a molecule of 30 to 50 kD molecular weight which increased glomerular permeability to plasma protein. The results, however, are questionable since the method used to size the molecule was exclusion chromatography. On her initial study she tested the factor in rats achieving proteinuria. However, when she attempted to further characterize the factor, she did not test the different fractions for protein excretion in the experimental animal but only for the presence of what she calls vascular permeability factor in an *in vitro* system. As we will show later, it is not proven that the *in vitro* test correlates with proteinuria in patients known to have the circulating factor.

Dantal group using sodium dodecyl sulfate polyacrylamide gel electrophoresis identified a band of 43 kD, likely to correspond to the vascular permeability factor reported by Savin as orosomucoid. When the purified orosomucoid was injected into rats, no differences were found between the proteinuria induced by the administration of the molecule from FSGS, non FSGS patients, and healthy individuals.

Savin and Dantal have described an *in vitro* test using isolated glomeruli to test for the presence of the factor that increases glomerular permeability. When the glomeruli are incubated in hypoosmotic medium and serum of some of these patients, the authors have observed that the glomerular volume increased but not as much as in controls. The difference was slight; only a 3% to 8% change in volume. The authors, then, have postulated that a factor in the serum of these patients increases the glomerular permeability to the proteins present in the capillary lumen and thus there is a decrease in the intraluminal oncotic pressure. Because of that, less water flows into the capillary lumen. The reliability and technical difficulties of the method are apparent in the frequency the factor is detected in patients with FSGS. From a high of 87% to 67% and only 25% in other studies.

What is the relationship between the noticed effect on glomerular volume and the increased glomerular capillary permeability to plasma proteins?

The effect on glomerular volume has been shown by Savin to be also induced by platelet derived growth factor (PDGF), tumor necrosis factor α (TNFα), and transforming growth factor β (TGFβ). However, none of these cytokines have been demonstrated to induce proteinuria when injected into rats. Therefore, the effect may be caused by a mechanism other than increased glomerular permeability to plasma proteins.

A cause-effect relationship between the circulating factor and the patient's proteinuria has not been established. After plasmapheresis, in Savin experience, "the proteinuria almost always reappeared within two weeks, whereas the factor was not rapidly synthesized after its removal, returning to the basal level only three months later". Attempts to correlate the presence of the factor detected using the *in vitro* test to proteinuria have shown mixed results. The correlation has been present when small sample population has been studied. No such correlation has been observed when a large sample has been studied. Moreover, there is a large overlap between nephrotic and controls and the definition of the presence or absence of the factor is arbitrary.

Factors present in supernatants of mononuclear cells cultures from LN patients

Supernatant factor isolated, effect on proteinuria [5]

In 1991, Koyama *et al.* developed a T cell hybridoma fusing lymphocytes from LN patients in relapse with a specific cell line. When the hybridoma supernatant were injected into rats, the urinary protein excretion, on the first day after injections, was significantly higher in rats injected hybridoma supernatant from LN patients as compared with rats infused hybridoma supernatant from normal controls.

Unfortunately, no further studies on the subject have been published since 1991 and thus there are no data on further characterization of the factor, of its presence in the serum of patients in relapse or in other glomerulopathies. Moreover, Dantal *et al.* were unable to reproduce the results.

Circulating factor isolated from serum and from supernatant of PBMC cultures. Factor identified. Proteinuria induced in the experimental animal. Effect abolished by the use of antibody against identified cytokine [6]

We have studied the effects of factor isolated from the supernatant of cultured PBMC from LN patients in relapse on rats glomerular heparan sulfate (GHS) and albuminuria. The factor was infused for 5 days using chronic catheterization of the left renal artery and an osmotic pump.

Prior to infusion, no differences in albumin excretion were found between rats to be infused with the fraction from patients in relapse and those to be infused with fraction from patients in remission, which served as controls. A significant increase in albuminuria was found on the 5th day of infusion compared with albuminuria prior to infusion when supernatant fraction from patients in relapse was used. No such effect was observed when the supernatant fraction from patients in remission was administered.

Because proteinuria in LN has been shown to be charge-dependent, we proceed to study the catabolism of the GHS in rats infused with supernatant factor from patients in relapse or infused with BSA used as controls. We studied the t 1/2 life of the GHS glycosaminoglycans (GAG) *in vivo* using standard pulse-chase technique. In rats infused with supernatant factor from patients in relapse, the t 1/2 life of the GHS GAG was markedly reduced suggesting that the primary effect of the factor is to increase the catabolism of the GHS GAG.

Identification of IL8 as the supernatant factor

Barratt *et al.* and we have observed a significantly increase in IL8 concentration in the supernatant of cultured PBMC and seruum of patients in relapse compared with LN patients in remission and normal control.

When IL8 was infused into rats at the average concentration of total IL8 present in the pooled supernatant of PBMC cultures from patients in relapse from our previous report, we observed a significant increase in urinary albumin/creatinine ratio on the 5th day of infusion compared with prior to infusion. No such changes were observed when BSA was infused. At the same time, we saw a significant decrease in glomerular heparan sulfate t 1/2 life in the left kidney infused with IL8 (26 h) compared with the t 1/2 in kidneys infused BSA alone (40 h).

Finally, when the supernatant factor was infused into rats with or without anti-IL8 neutralizing antibody, there was a significant increase in albuminuria on the last day of infusion compared with prior to infusion when supernatant factor was infused alone. No such differences in albumin excretion were found on the 5th day of infusion when same supernatant factor and the addition of anti-IL8 antibody were used. Moreover, when anti-IL8 was added to the supernatant factor, the effect on sulfate uptake by the supernatant on the GBM was abolished.

IL8, therefore, may play a role in the pathogenesis of MC nephrotic syndrome by increasing the catabolism of the GHS GAG. As a result, the glomerular charge barrier is reduced and there is an increase in permeability to plasma proteins.

In summary, despite all our efforts we cannot define yet the nature of the circulating factor in these diseases. The search for these factors and their mechanism for the proteinuria will be enhanced if more is known about glomerular filtration physiology. Finally, we will not find a definitive answer regarding this factor unless there is a combined effort to standardize the methodology to isolate, characterize, and infuse the factor into the experimental animal.

References

1. Levin M, Smith C, Walters MDS, Gascoine P, Barratt M. Steroid-responsive nephrotic syndrome: a generalized disorder of membrane negative charge. *Lancet* 1985; II: 239-42.
2. Bakker WW, Baller JFW, van Luijk WHJ. A kallikrein-like molecule and plasma vaso-activity in minimal change disease. *Contrib Nephrol* 1988; 67: 1-36.
3. Sharma M, Sharma R, McCarthy ET, Savin VJ. "The FSGS factor": enrichment and *in vivo* effect of activity from focal segmental glomerulosclerosis plasma. *J Am Soc Nephrol* 1999; 10: 552-61.
4. Le Berre L, Godfrin Y, Lafond-Puyet L, Perretto S, Le Carrer D, Bouhours JF, Soulillou JP, Dantal J. Effect of plasma fractions from patients with focal and segmental glomerulosclerosis on rat proteinuria. *Kidney Int* 2000; 58: 2502-11.
5. Koyama A, Fuhsaki M, Kobayashi M, Igarashi M, Narita M. A glomerular permeability factor produced by human T-cell hybridomas. *Kidney Int* 1991; 40: 453-60.
6. Garin EH, Laflam P, Chandler L.Anti-interleukin 8 antibody abolishes effects of lipoid nephrosis cytokine. *Pediatr Nephrol* 1998; 12: 381-5.

Recurrence of the Disease in the Renal Graft
Cochat P, ed.
© John Libbey Eurotext, Paris, 2001

A practical approach to the prediction of recurrence of focal segmental glomerulosclerosis in renal allograft recipients

Nicholas J.A. Webb
Royal Manchester Children's Hospital, Manchester, United Kingdom

Since Hoyer *et al.*'s first description of recurrence of focal segmental glomerulosclerosis (FSGS) in a renal allograft recipient [1], there have been a significant number of publications reporting series of both children and adults with recurrent disease, including reports from both individual transplant centres and transplant registries. This manuscript aims to discuss the proposed risk factors for recurrent FSGS in the transplanted kidney with the aim of providing a guide to patient management, in particular to assist in the counselling of patients with FSGS prior to transplantation regarding the risk of them developing recurrent disease. The understanding of the risk factors for disease recurrence additionally allows the physician to target research investigating the aetiology of recurrent disease.

Proposed risk factors for recurrent disease to be discussed include: i) duration of disease from onset to development of end stage renal failure (ESRF), ii) race, iii) disease recurrence in a previous transplant, iv) the presence of mesangial proliferation in the original native renal biopsy, v) age at initial diagnosis, vi) donor source and degree of HLA matching, vii) immunosuppressive therapy and viii) time on dialysis prior to transplantation. These will be discussed individually.

As the number of individuals with a primary diagnosis of FSGS undergoing renal transplantation is relatively small, and the number of these developing recurrent diseases even smaller, small and moderate sized series from individual centres may be underpowered to confirm or refute the validity of postulated risk factors for disease recurrence. Only larger registry series are likely to be appropriately powered. Comparison of the results of series from different centres is made difficult by great variety in the ethnicity of the population under study, with some North American series consisting of a large proportion of African Americans and Hispanics in whom FSGS is more prevalent and possibly behaves differently. Other difficulties encountered in comparing studies is that some include only those patients with clinical evidence of recurrent nephrotic syndrome and histological changes of FSGS in the graft [2], whereas others make the diagnosis solely on the detection of heavy proteinuria [3]. In some series, patients are included who have previously been reported in earlier publications from the same centre [2, 4].

Overall, the reported incidence of recurrent FSGS, based on paediatric registry data, is 21% (95%CI 14-27%) in North America [5] and 29% in Europe [6], though smaller series from single centres report a rate of between 5.6% [7] and 100% [8]. As discussed above, some variability in incidence may be accounted for by differences in the diagnosis of disease recurrence. Recurrent FSGS is clearly a large clinical problem. The EDTA registry, reporting graft losses secondary to recurrent disease between 1980 and 1991 found that 24% of kidneys lost in patients under 15 years of age with FSGS were attributable to recurrent disease [9]. Adult registry data show that the relative risk of graft failure because of recurrent FSGS is 2.25 (1.6-3.1) [10].

Duration of disease from onset to development of ESRF

There is almost complete uniformity in reported series in the detection of a short time from disease presentation to the development of ESRF as a risk factor for disease recurrence. In the large North American Pediatric Renal Transplant Co-operative Study (NAPRTCS) registry series of Tejani and Stablein, the mean time from diagnosis to ESRF was 33 months in those with recurrence and 52 months in those without [5]. Whilst the EDTA did not collect data on primary disease duration, the NAPRTCS findings are replicated almost without exception in single centre reports. In Europe, Wuhl et al. found the mean interval from diagnosis to ESRF was 3.0 years in relapsing patients compared with 7.9 years in non-relapsing patients [3] and similar findings were reported by Dall'Amico et al. (3.9 years vs 6.2 years) [11] and Senggutuvan et al. (3.5 vs 5.0 yrs) [4]. In North America, Striegel et al. also found time from diagnosis to ESRF of less than 3 years to be a significant risk factor for recurrent disease; those with recurrent disease had a mean time to ESRF of 2.8 years compared with 5.5 years for those with no recurrence [2]. Only Ingulli and Tejani, reporting a predominantly African American and Hispanic population from New York, failed to detect a similar finding, perhaps reflecting the difference in the natural history of the disease in these ethic groups as discussed later [12].

These paediatric data are supported by data from adult patients. Dantal et al., reporting a large series from Nantes, found a mean disease duration of 64.5 ± 16.4 months in relapsing patients compared with 132 ± 19.6 months in the non-relapsing recipients [13].

Race

In North American series, African American race has been shown to be protective against the development of recurrent disease. Tejani and Stablein reporting NAPRTCS data found a 9% recurrence rate amongst African Americans compared with 23% in Whites and 20% in Hispanic patients [5]. Butani et al. recently reported a series of 27 transplants performed in a single centre and also found recurrence to occur less frequently in African Americans compared with Caucasian children, though this did not reach statistical significance [14]. These findings perhaps go some way to explain the variation between previous studies from single centres in the reported incidence of recurrent disease, with Ingulli and Tejani reporting a recurrence rate of 15% in a predominantly African American population from New York [12] and Striegel et al. reporting a rate of 50% in a predominantly White population from Minnesota [2].

No series from European centres have reported data on ethnicity.

Disease recurrence in a previous transplant

The number of patients undergoing retransplantation following recurrent disease is relatively small, though a number of observations strongly suggest that recurrence after primary transplantation places the subsequent graft at increased risk. This subject has probably been best investigated by Stephanian et al. who studied the outcome of 22 retransplants in 14 adult patients [15]. Of the 6 patients who lost their first graft to rejection, none developed recurrent disease in the subsequent graft, whereas of the 8 who lost their first graft to recurrent disease, 6 had recurrences in a total of 10 out of 14 subsequent transplants. Furthermore, first graft longevity appeared to be linked to subsequent recurrence risk: the 3 patients who lost their subsequent grafts to recurrent disease had much earlier loss of their primary graft (2-13 months) than those who maintained reasonable function in their subsequent grafts (47-126 months). Dantal et al. found that recurrence occurred in 75-80% of second grafts where this had occurred after the first transplant [13].

Similar observations have been made in paediatric series. Striegel et al. reported 10 children undergoing retransplantation and noted that none of the 6 patients who lost their graft for other reasons developed FSGS in their subsequent graft in contrast to 3 out of 4 with graft loss secondary to FSGS who developed recurrent disease upon retransplantation [2]. The EDTA registry reported a 27% recurrence rate after first transplantation, with this rate increasing to 36% after second transplantation: of 7 children who showed a recurrence after their first transplant, 6 also developed recurrent disease after their second graft [16].

Presence of mesangial proliferation in the native renal biopsy

The presence of mesangial proliferation superimposed upon the pathological lesion of FSGS in the native kidney has been proposed as a risk factor for recurrent disease by a number of authors reporting series from individual centres following an early report by Maizel et al. [17]. Striegel et al. reported a series of 37 transplants in 24 patients transplanted with a primary diagnosis of FSGS [2]. Recurrences occurred after 16 transplants in 12 patients. Careful review of the native renal biopsies was performed, and patients were classified as having "pure" FSGS (n = 10), FSGS with mild mesangial proliferation (n = 8) and FSGS with diffuse mesangial proliferation (n = 6). Recurrence rates for the three groups were 11.6%, 60% and 80% respectively, supporting the presence of mesangial proliferation as a significant risk factor. Similarly, in Europe, Senggutuvan et al., reporting from Guys Hospital found mesangial prominence to be a significant risk factor, being present in 10 out of 11 recipients with recurrence and 12 out of 22 without, though separate analysis of paediatric and adult recipients showed that this finding was restricted to paediatric patients [4]. Registry data do not, however, support the findings of these smaller series: Tejani and Stablein did not detect any difference in recurrence rate between those with mesangial proliferation (25%) and those without (20%) [5] and the EDTA registry data reported by Rizzoni et al. also failed to find the presence of mesangial proliferation to be predictive of recurrence [6]. There may, of course, be some variability in the detail with which the presence and extent of mesangial hypercellularity is reported between centres contributing to registry data. It remains unclear as to whether FSGS with diffuse MP is the result of a different disease process from that which results in "pure" FSGS.

Striegel et al. suggested that the presence of mesangial proliferation and time from initial diagnosis to the development of to ESRF were linked as risk factors for recurrence, in that those patients who had a rapid decline into ESRF were also more likely to have mesangial proliferation on their biopsy [2].

Age at initial diagnosis

Whilst a number of reports have suggested that young age at initial diagnosis of FSGS is a risk factor for disease recurrence, these have generally been those which included both adult and paediatric patients [4]. There appears to be little dispute that children experience disease recurrence more frequently than adults. Analysis of paediatric data fails to detect a link between age at first diagnosis and recurrence risk. The NAPRTCS series did not find any difference in recurrence rates with differing age at initial diagnosis [5], and this finding was also observed in a number of single centre series [2, 4, 11]. The EDTA registry data, however, reporting on 39 recurrences showed a recurrence rate of 17% in those up to 6 years of age and 40% in those older than 6 years [6], with this finding also being replicated in a single centre study [3]. Only Ingulli and Tejani have found young age to be a risk factor for disease recurrence in a relatively small series of almost exclusively Black and Hispanic children: the older age at presentation and lower relapse rate in the African American population may have influenced this finding [12].

Donor source and degree of HLA matching

A number of early reports suggested that recurrence of FSGS was more common in well-matched grafts and commoner in living-related donor kidneys than cadaveric. The NAPRTCS data did not confirm this finding, with recurrence being similar (18% cadaveric and 24% LRD). Furthermore, two-year graft survival was statistically significantly superior following LRD transplantation (64% vs 74%, p<0.05) [5]. Similarly, more recent large series from Europe have also found no difference in outcome [4]. EDTA Registry data have failed to show any link between recurrence rate and either donor source or degree of HLA matching [16]. Whilst some have suggested that living donors should not be used in patients with FSGS in view of the significant risk of graft loss from recurrent disease, Tejani and Stablein commented that the improved graft survival did not justify such an approach being taken [5].

Immunosuppressive therapy

Despite a number of early speculative reports, there appears to be no firm evidence that the introduction of calcineurin inhibitors and other more modern immunosuppressive agents has resulted in an improvement in disease recurrence rates. One recent study by Raafat et al. has suggested that the introduction of polyclonal antibodies as induction agents has resulted in an increase in recurrence rate [18].

Time on dialysis prior to transplantation

Despite suggestions that a prolonged period of dialysis prior to transplantation might reduce the recurrence rate through improved clearance of circulating factors responsible for disease recurrence, most series fail to show any effect of dialysis duration and no useful purpose appears to be served in keeping the patient on protracted dialysis therapy [2, 4, 5].

Conclusions

In conclusion, there appears to be reasonable evidence that a short duration from diagnosis to the development of ESRF, non-African American race (in North America), disease recurrence in a previous transplant and disease presentation in childhood are risk factors for recurrent FSGS following transplantation. Some evidence supports the presence of mesangial hypercellularity in the native renal biopsy as a risk factor. Donor source, immunosuppressive therapy and time on dialysis prior to transplantation appear to have no influence on outcome.

References

1. Hoyer JR, Raij L, Vernier RL, Simmons RL, Najarian JS, Michael AF. Recurrence of idiopathic nephrotic syndrome after renal transplantation. *Lancet* 1972; 2: 343.
2. Striegel JE, Sibley RK, Fryd DS, Mauer SM. Recurrence following focal segmental sclerosis in children following renal transplantation. *Kidney Int* 1986; 30: S44-9.
3. Wuhl E, Frdryk J, Wiesel M, Mehls O, Schaefer F, Scharer K. Impact of recurrent nephrotic syndrome after renal transplantation in young patients. *Pediatr Nephrol* 1998; 12: 529-33.
4. Senggutuvan P, Cameron JS, Hartley RB, Rigden S, Chantler C, Haycock G, Williams DG, Ogg C, Koffman G. Recurrence of focal segmental glomerulosclerosis in transplanted kidneys: analysis of incidence and risk factors in 59 allografts. *Pediatr Nephrol* 1990; 4: 21-8.
5. Tejani A, Stablein DH. Recurrence of focal segmental glomerulosclerosis posttransplantation: a special report of the North American Pediatric Renal Transplant Co-operative Study. *J Am Soc Nephrol* 1992; 2: S258-63.
6. Rizzoni G, Ehrich JHH, Brunner FP, Geerlings W, Fassbinder W, Landais P, Mallick N, Margreiter R, Raine AEG, Selwood NH, Tufveson G. Combined report on regular dialysis and transplantation of children in Europe 1990. *Nephrol Dial Transplant* 1991; 6: S31-42.
7. Malekzadeh MH, Houser ET, Ettenger RB, et al.. Focal glomerulosclerosis and renal transplantation. *J Pediatr* 1979; 95: 249-51.
8. Alexsen RA, Seymour AE, Mathew TH, Fisher G, Canny A, Pascoe V. Recurrent focal glomerulosclerosis in renal transplants. *Clin Nephrol* 1984; 21: 110-2.

9. Briggs JD, Jones E. Recurrence of glomerulonephritis following renal transplantation.*Nephrol Dial Transplant* 1999; 14: 564-5.
10. Hariharan S, Adams MB, Brennan DC, Davis CL, First MR, Johnson CP, Ouseph R, Peddi VR, Pelz CL, Roza AM, Vincenti F, George V. Recurrent and de novo glomerular disease after renal transplantation.
11. Dall'Amico R, Ghiggeri G, Carraro M, Artero M, Ghio L, Zamorani E, Zennaro C, Basile G, Montino G, Rivabella L, Cardillo M, Scalamonga M, Ginevri F. Prediction and treatment of recurrent focal segmental glomerulosclerosis after renal transplantation in children. *Am J Kid Dis* 1999; 34: 1048-55.
12. Ingulli E, Tejani A. Incidence, treatment, and outcome of recurrent focal segmental glomerulosclerosis posttransplantation in 42 allografts in children: a single centre experience. *Transplantation* 1991; 51: 401-5.
13. Dantal J, Soulillou JP. Relapse of focal segmental glomerulosclerosis after kidney transplantation. *Adv Nephrol* 1996; 25: 91-106.
14. Butani L, Polinski MS, Kaiser BA, Baluarte HJ. Predictive value of race in post-transplantation recurrence of focal segmental glomerulosclerosis in children. *Nephrol Dial Transplant* 1999; 14: 166-8.
15. Stephanian E, Matas AJ, Mauer M, Chavers B, Nevins T, Kashtan C, Sutherland DER, Gores P, Najarian JS. Recurrence of disease in patients retransplanted for focal segmental glomerulosclerosis. *Transplantation* 1992; 53: 755-7.
16. Ehrich JHH, Loirat C, Brunner FP, Geerlings W, Landais P, Mallick NP, Margreiter R, Raine AEG, Selwood NH, Tufveson G, Valderrabano F. Report on management of renal failure in children in Europe. XXII, 1991. *Nephrol Dial Transplant* 1992; (Suppl. 2): 36-48.
17. Maizel S, Sibley RK, Houstman JP, Kjellsatrand CM, Simmons RL. Incidence and significance of recurrent focal and segmental glomerulosclerosis in renal allograft recipients. *Transplantation* 1981; 32: 512-6.
18. Raafat R, Travis LB, Kalia A, Diven S. Role of transplant induction therapy on recurrence rate of focal segmental glomerulosclerosis. *Pediatr Nephrol* 2000; 14: 189-94.

Plasma treatments for patients with recurrence of focal segmental glomerular sclerosis after renal transplantation

Dan Hristea, Ludmilla Le Berre, Claude Guyot, Maryvonne Hourmant, Jean-Paul Soulillou, Jacques Dantal

Institut de Transplantation et de Recherche en Transplantation (ITERT) and Institut National de la Santé et de la Recherche Médicale (INSERM), Unit 437, CHU Hôtel-Dieu, Nantes, France

After renal transplantation, 30 to 50% of patients with idiopathic nephrotic syndrome (INS) and focal glomerulosclerosis (FSGS) experience relapse of proteinuria (see [1] for review). The occurrence of such immediate relapse has for a long time suggested that some patients with INS and/or FSGS possess a circulating factor(s) capable of altering glomerular permeability in a normal graft [2, 3]. Evidence for the presence of a putative plasmatic factor was first sustained by the demonstration of an increased urinary protein excretion in rats after infusion with sera from an FSGS patient with recurrence after transplantation [4]. Similar results were reported following injection of plasmatic fractions [5] and protein A eluats [6] but the transfer of albuminuric activity to rats is a difficult and disputed model [7]. On such a basis, plasma treatment appears to be a logical method of treating FSGS recurrence. Plasmapheresis has been reported as having mixed results in several series of patients [8-11]. In the present study, we report the efficacy of plasma treatment in treating recurrence of nephrotic syndrome in renal transplant recipients.

Patients, material and methods

Definition of recurrence

Clinical diagnosis of recurrent FSGS was made in the case of rapid onset of selective proteinuria after transplantation in a patient having biopsy proven FSGS as the cause of primary renal failure. Proteinuria exceeding 1 g/day was defined as the time of onset of recurrence. In all cases, a renal biopsy was performed in order to exclude acute rejection and to confirm recurrence. Biopsy evidence of either effacement of epithelial foot processes *via* electron microscopy and/or focal segmental lesions *via* light microscopy were considered compatible with the diagnosis of recurrence. The existence of FSGS lesions as seen by an early biopsy was not mandatory for diagnosis.

Patients

We reviewed the files of all patients who received plasmapheresis or immuno-adsorption treatment for recurrent FSGS between January 1985 and April 2001 in the nephrology unit of the University Hospital in Nantes. During this period, 2,145 renal transplantations were performed. Among these, the cause of renal failure was FSGS in 105 patients (4.9%) and 25 patients (24%) had recurrence of nephrotic syndrome after transplantation. Four additional patients from other transplantation centers were referred for immunoadsorption. These 29 patients received a total of 31 transplants. The age of the patients at the time of onset of clinical disease ranged from 24 months to 50 years, with an average of 22.8 ± 15.9 years. Eighteen patients were male and 11 were female. The management of the primary INS varied, all patients had received at least one course of standard steroid therapy. Thirteen patients received one course of an alkylating agent (chlorambucil, n = 5, cyclophosphamide, n = 8) or azathioprine (2 patients) usually in combination with steroids. In addition, 8 patients received cyclosporin A. The interval between the onset of clinical disease and ESRF ranged from 1 to 19 years with a median of 46 months.

Patient age at transplantation ranged from 9.8 to 67.3 years (median 27.2 years), 5 patients were under 15 years of age at the time of transplantation. All grafts were of cadaver origin. Nine patients received a second graft and one a third. For these latter patients, the first transplanted organ underwent FSGS recurrence with a mean graft survival of 2.4 ± 1.9 years. Two patients transplanted in our unit have both their first and the second graft included in this study.

During the study period we used different immunosuppressive regimens. Briefly, from 1985 to 1995, first transplanted FSGS recipients received a sequential quadruple therapy of ATG (Imtix-Sangstat, France), azathioprine, prednisone and cyclosporin A and from 1995, either CsA or FK506, MMF and prednisone. A total of 24 transplantations were undertaken with ATG given during 11.2 ± 3.4 days and 4 with an anti-IL2R antibody (Simulect, Novartis). The main maintenance therapy used was CsA-AZA (25 patients), in addition, the remaining patients received either CsA-MMF (3 patients) or FK506-MMF (3 patients).

Our policy for the treatment of recurrence was firstly to the reinforcement of immunosuppression by increasing blood concentrations of cyclosporine A or FK506 to trough levels above 250 ng/ml and 15 ng/ml respectively. In the case of persistent proteinuria (*i.e.* > 3 g/d), patients were included in a plasmapheresis or immunoadsorption treatment protocol without any further modification of the immunosuppressive treatment. For three pediatric patients, the protocol described by P. Cochat was used where, in addition to plasmapheresis, 3 pulses of steroids were administered and AZA replaced by cyclophosphamide [12]. The introduction of ACE-inhibitors, AT2 antagonists or statins treatments was allowed after a first series of plasma treatment, otherwise these therapies remained unmodified during phase I *(see below)*.

Plasma exchange (PE)

Plasmapheresis procedures were performed either by plasma filtration (PF2000, Gambro, Germany) or by centrifugation (BT798, Dideco, Italy or Cobe Spectra, France).

During each session (a one day procedure), a total of 50 ml/kg and/or a maximum of 4 liters were replaced with a saline solution supplemented with 4% albumin or for two patients by fresh frozen plasma. These sessions were repeated 5 to 10 times over 10 to 20 days (referred to as Phase I treatment). When treatment was successful, it was followed by a maintenance treatment of one PE session whenever proteinuria return to a threshold of 3 g/day (Phase II).

Plasma immunoadsorption (IA)

The plasma separation device delivers a continuous flow rate of plasma to a pair of immunoadsorption cartridges (Ig-Therasorb, Therasorb, Germany [13] or Protein A, Immunosorba, Excorim, Sweden [14]). The same pair of cartridges was used for the treatment of a single patient. The CITEM 10 (Excorim) or the ADA adsorption system (Therasorb) was used to monitor plasma flow as well as column washing and elution procedures at pH 2.8 (0.2 M glycine buffer). Immunoadsorption cartridges contained Protein A covalently linked to Sepharose (Immunosorba) or immobilized sheep antibodies specific for the heavy chains of human IgG and for the kappa and lambda chains (Ig-Therasorb). These pyrogen-free columns were stored at 4 °C until use.

IA treatment consisted of repeated one-day procedures (sessions) during which 2.5 plasma volumes were treated, the sessions being repeated 5 to 10 times over a period of 10 to 20 days (Phase I). After this Phase I treatment, intravenous immunoglobulins (IVIg, Endobulines, Austria) were injected according to the formula: IVIg = (IgG level before treatment x body weight) x 0.04. A further IA cycle was proposed if proteinuria remained above 3 g/day. Treatment, when successful, was followed by a "maintenance" IA treatment of 1 session whenever proteinuria return to a threshold of 3 g/day (Phase II).

Results

Effect of Phase I plasma treatment

A total of 41 Phase I treatments (23 PE and 18 IA) were carried out for 31 cases of recurrence. Three patients had two Phase I PE cycles, 6 patients had both PE and IA cycles and two patients had two Phase I IA cycles (protein A and Ig-Therasorb). All patients presented a recurrence of idiopathic nephrotic syndrome with a proteinuria above 1g/d after a median of 2 days (ranging from 1 to 90) and above 3 g/d after a median of 9 days post-transplantation (ranging from 1 to 550). The time of the initiation of the first Phase I treatment post-transplantation ranged from 12 to 707 days (median 60 days). Before treatment, proteinuria was at 11.2 ± 12 g/d (median 8.26), serum creatinine at 193 ± 123 µmol/l and CsA trough levels at 199 ± 100 ng/ml. A mean of 6.9 ± 2.4 sessions were performed per patient.

After the Phase I treatment, proteinuria was unaffected (remained above 3 g/d and/or decreased less than 50%) in 14 patients (failure rate of 33%, 10 in the PE group and 4 in the IA group), for the remaining patients proteinuria dropped after the Phase I treatment to 2.17 ± 2.69 ($76.5 \pm 18\%$ decrease) and 13 patients presented a proteinuria below 1g/d. There was a slight but non significant improvement in renal function after the Phase I treatment to 170 ± 97 µmol/l. The level of proteinuria and the presence of FSGS lesions in the kidney graft biopsy before treatment were the two parameters predictive of the efficacy of the Phase I treatment. In the responsive group, proteinuria was at 7.7 ± 4.8 g/d *versus* 20.25 ± 18 g/d in non responsive patients ($p < 0.002$) and FSGS lesions were present in 10% *versus* 71% of the pre-Phase I biopsies. With regards to these two factors, there was no difference when we compared the global response to PE and IA treatments. Nevertheless, when the two treatments were applied in the same patient, the IA (performed from 1 to 16 months after PE) had a more pronounced effect on proteinuria (decreased in proteinuria of $85 \pm 12\%$ *versus* $55 \pm 15\%$, $p < 0.02$) and induced a partial remission (from 6.6 to 1.2 g/d) in one patient while PE was unsuccessful. In addition, there was no difference in the effect of the two IA procedures (protein A *versus* Ig-Therasorb).

After Phase I treatment, a partial remission (reduction in the proteinuria to below 3 g/d and/or by more than 50% of the pre-treatment value) was obtained in 9 patients (5 PE and 4 IA) and a complete remission (proteinuria below 1 g/d) in 18 patients (10 PE and 8 IA). Nevertheless, a long lasting remission (for more than 6 months) was only achieved in 4 patients, in the others the proteinuria returned to above 3 g/d or to the pre-Phase I values within 16.6 ± 10 and 31 ± 25 days for patients with partial and complete remission, respectively.

Effect of Phase II plasma treatment

After Phase I, a chronic treatment (Phase II) was suggested whenever proteinuria returned to above 3 g/day. A total of 21 Phase II treatments were performed in 16 patients (8 PE and 13 IA). A mean of 10 sessions per patient were carried out and after each session a mild but significant decrease of proteinuria from 6.4 ± 4 to 4.1 ± 3.4 g/day (mean of decrease of $47.6 \pm 22\%$) was induced. The mean interval between two sessions was 16.7 ± 6.8 days, ranging from 7 to 27 days. This chronic treatment was interrupted in all but 2 patients (still on PE) either due to failure to maintain proteinuria below 3 g/d (7 patients), loss of efficacy (5 patients after 6 to 26 sessions), removal of consent, technical reasons (4 patients) or for 3 patients due to a remission with a proteinuria below 1 g/d.

Overall effect of plasmatic treatment on graft survival

Graft survival is presented in *Figure 1*. Without response to Phase I treatment, the survival rate was no more than 50% 2 years post-transplantation with a significantly better graft survival for the responder group ($p < 0.03$). There was no impact of the type of plasma treatment on the graft survival (PE *versus* IA) whatever the response. Five of 26 adult patients showed a long lasting remission with a proteinuria below 1 g for at least 6 months. Their grafts are all functional and one patient showed a chronic rejection pattern 13 years after transplantation. All three pediatric patients included in the protocol described by P. Cochat also showed a long lasting remission with, in two of them, a recurrence treated again with success by the same strategy. Only a few non life-threating, adverse events occurred during the treatment period (one bleeding and

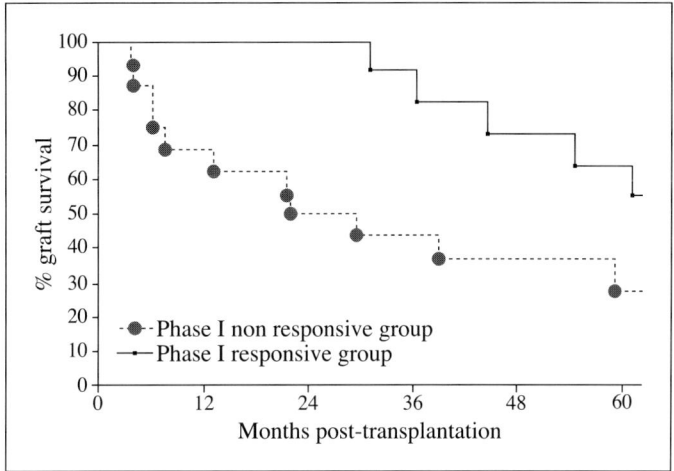

Figure 1. Graft survival (Kaplan Meir) of patients with FSGS recurrence after renal transplantation according to the response to Phase I plasma treatment.

two technical problems concerning venous access, one hypocalcemia, and one allergic reaction to albumin). We also observed one pneumonia but no other events related to over-immunosuppression. Finally, one patient developed a severe pancreatitis while undergoing in Phase II treatment. This treatment maintained proteinuria below 3 g/d but cessation of immunoadsorption was followed by a dramatic worsening of the daily protcinuria to up to 25 g.

Discussion

Considering the high reported rate of graft loss in kidney transplant patients with recurrent proteinuria due to recurrent FSGS, a rational and effective strategy is required. Different therapies have been proposed to treat these patients including non-steroid anti-inflammatory drugs [15], angiotensin converting enzyme inhibitors [16], high dose cyclosporin [17] and plasma treatment by PE [8-10, 18-20] or immunoadsorption [6, 21, 22]. The mechanisms underlying idiopathic nephrotic syndrome are still not understood and are probably multiple. The group of patients with FSGS recurrence after renal transplantation is probably more homogeneous. The observations of 1) immediate recurrence after transplantation, 2) the remission of proteinuria after transplantation of a proteinuric kidney into a "normal environment" [23, 24] and 3) the results of an *in vitro* assay which detects permeability changes induced by recurrent FSGS serum on isolated glomeruli [25, 26] strongly suggest the presence of a plasmatic factor that triggers a rapid alteration of glomerular permeability. These observations support the hypothesis that plasma treatment could be an efficacious treatment modality for these patients. However, the success of PE has been reported with variable results in small series of patients. Since the first single case reports of successful PE [4, 27], there has been during the last decade an increased number of short series that confirm the interest of PE, particularly for pediatric patients [18-20].

Our series of 31 recurrent FSGS patients treated by PE/IA is, to our knowledge, the largest to be reported in the literature. According to our previous experience, the results of PE and IA treatments are mixed and demonstrate a similar efficacy. Several conclusions can be drawn from the literature and from our series. Firstly, the effect of PE/IA on the reduction in proteinuria correlates with its pre-treatment level. Secondly, the observation of FSGS lesions at the time of the PE/IA is usually associated with treatment failure. Thirdly, although not seen in our cohort of patients, the efficacy of PE/IA seems to correlate with its early initiation after transplantation. Fourthly, in adult patients, the remission of proteinuria is transient with a return to pre-treatment values within 1 month. Finally, IA seems to induce a more profound effect on proteinuria than PE, but the response rate is similar and only a few patients achieve long lasting remission (19% lasting more than 6 months). In the other reported series, PE is performed, immediately following diagnosis of recurrence, with modifications of immunosuppression which can change, *per se*, the evolution of the outcome of recurrence. Nevertheless, in pediatric patients, the combination of corticosteroid boluses, cyclophosphamide and high-doses of CsA, has been shown to induce an excellent rate of long lasting remission [12, 18] and an additional effect or a synergy of these treatments with PE/IA can be supposed. In our study, an effect of the high intravenous doses of immunoglobulins (IVIg) can be ruled out as proteinuria in our patients clearly fell before the administration of IVIg. Furthermore, IVIg were found to be inefficient in reducing albuminuria in a short series of pediatric cases of idiopathic nephrotic syndrome [28].

However, the efficacy of PE/IA must be interpreted cautiously as the studies were not conducted in a prospective fashion and the number of patients is small. The very early initiation of PE/IA seems to be a key factor in the success but this can be misinterpreted as remission can be observed after the introduction of immunosuppressive drugs, especially CsA [17] or spontaneously [29]. On the other hand, the interest for chronic plasma treatment is difficult to assess. In our series, this regimen was able to maintain the proteinuria below the nephrotic range, thus improving the clinical tolerance to the recurrence. A positive impact on graft survival was expected but not demonstrated and the occurrence of chronic vascular lesions could participate in the failure of this chronic treatment (late loss of efficacy).

Our results in adults, in terms of long lasting remission, are poor and are contrary to the results reported in children. It is not clear whether idiopathic nephrotic syndrome in children and adults is the same entity but some parameters could explain this failure. The threshold of the selective proteinuria at 3 g/d for the initiation of PE/IA is probably too high. Some patients present a low aggressive disease or a recurrence partially controlled by CsA, at the beginning of the transplantation that could, in this strategy, delay the onset of the PE/IA to a less favorable condition (*i.e.* glomerular damage). We stopped the PE/IA treatment after 5 to 10 sessions in the case of unresponsiveness ; however, recent publications suggest maintaining this therapy for a prolonged period because of a gradual response. According to the low number of patients, only a multicentric study will help a more efficient protocol to be defined. We modified our strategy with initiation of PE/IA as soon as the selective proteinuria reached 1 g/day (with Cyp introduction in the case of a non-response) and in the absence of complications, for a systematic 6 month Phase II treatment.

The possibility of an imbalance between permeability factors and their inhibitors has also been postulated in the literature [30]. We have tested this hypothesis by comparing the substitution by fresh frozen plasma with albumin. Until now, only two patients have been analyzed during Phase II treatment without any differences between the two substitutions.

The nature of the factor removed by PE/IA remains elusive. The analysis of the plasmapheretic fluid offers the opportunity to perform different *in vitro* and *in vivo* studies. Savin *et al.* were the first to use this fluid in fractionation experiments using the ammonium sulfate (AS) precipitation technique, and have shown, *via* their *in vitro* assay of glomerular permeability, that the albuminuric activity was only detected in the 70-80% AS precipitate fraction [25]. After injection into rat, this fraction induced a significant increase in proteinuria when compared to the fraction from normal controls [5]. Its molecular mass was estimated to be approximately 50 kD and it was suggested to be a non-immunoglobulin protein or a fragment of an immunoglobulin [21]. However, there might be traces of autoantibodies-directed, for instance, against podocyte antigens - which would be sufficient to trigger a signal leading to albuminuria although produced at a concentration too low to be immunologically detected. We have also tested the *in vivo* effect of Ig-depleted fractions obtained from PE in rats and demonstrated that the induction of proteinuria is not significantly different from the control fractions [7]. Despite some differences on SDS-PAGE analysis, we were unable to characterize the albuminuric factor and the rat is probably not a reliable model of this disease.

In conclusion, it is suggested that PE/IA could be an effective form of treatment for FSGS recurrence after transplantation but needs further optimization through multicentric large cohorts of patients. If started early, proteinuria can be substantially reduced and/or maintained to a low level by repeated sessions. Nevertheless, these results must be interpreted cautiously due to the small number of patients, especially adult patients, and the impact of these treatments on long term graft survival has not yet been demonstrated.

Acknowledgments

We are grateful to Pr. Bourbigot (Brest), Pr. Lebranchu (Tours), Pr Hurault de Ligny (Caen) and Pr. Noel (Lille) for referring patients with immediate recurrence of INS after transplantation to us and to Joanna Ashton for editing the manuscript.

This work was supported in part by a 1996 Baxter Extramural Grant, by a grant from the PHRC (95/5J) and by the Fondation Transvie.

References

1. Senggutuvan P, Cameron JS, Hartley RB, Riggen S, Chantler C, Williams DG, Ogg C, Koffman G. Recurrence of focal segmental glomerulosclerosis in transplanted kidneys: analysis of incidence and risk factors in 59 allografts. *Pediatr Nephrol* 1990; 4: 21-8.

positive with gradual decline of the GFR. Stage V is end stage renal disease (ESRD) that is characterized by minimal residual renal function requiring dialysis. The usual time between diabetes onset and ESRD is from 20 to 30 years.

Whether glycemic control determines the rates of progression or amelioration of the structural and functional abnormalities of diabetic nephropathy in humans was a major research question. Data from animals [6] demonstrated that islet transplantation or optimum insulin treatment altered the course of the structural and functional lesions of diabetic renal disease. In man several studies [7, 8] such as Diabetes Control and Complications Trial (DCCT) demonstrated quite convincingly that euglycemia affected the development and/or the progression of human renal disease. Structural and functional lesions of diabetic nephropathy evolve over the first 2-3 decades of disease: the increase in GBM width becomes evident during the first 10 years followed by a measurable expansion of mesangium and microalbuminuria during the second decade of disease. In order to alter the course of albuminuria in the DCCT, five or more years of lowered hemoglobin A1c were necessary before a clear benefit of intensive management became apparent. Steffes [8] demonstrated clearly that early histologic lesions could be beneficially altered by the establishment of euglycemia.

Thus, intensive glycemic control can modify functional and structural manifestations of diabetic nephropathy and a period of about a decade is necessary before any clear benefit may be demonstrated.

Alterations of the glomerular structure in renal allografts when grafted in patients with insulin-dependent diabetes

Recurrent diabetic nephropathy is an important cause of graft dysfunction and eventual loss. Mauer *et al.* [9] were the first to describe hyaline arteriosclerosis in renal transplantations of diabetic patients within 5 years after transplantation. Osterby in 1991 [10] used in these patients the same morphometric analysis employed to study the early stages of diabetic nephropathy. She showed that 2 or 3 years after transplantation in kidney grafts the mean value of GBM thickness was about 55 nm and the mesangial volume was 22% wider than that reported in kidneys grafted in non-diabetic subjects. In diabetic patients who receive conventional insulin therapy, thickening of the GBM can be detected in renal allografts after only 2 years at rates of change similar to those in native kidneys of newly diagnosed diabetic patients. Although the rate of change in the thickness of GBM varies among patients, it remains remarkably constant in individual patients evaluated 2 and 5 years after renal transplantation. The Minneapolis group [9, 11] as well as the Stockolm group [10, 12] showed that the increase in the relative mesangial volume in renal allografts was as early as 2 years after transplantation. These data suggested that mesangial widening may develop more rapidly in recurrent transplant diabetic nephropathy than in diabetic patient's own kidneys. The same groups from Minneapolis [13] and Stockolm [12] suggested the existence of two groups of diabetic renal transplant recipients with regard to the light microscopic changes: one group showing only slight changes after several years after transplantation and the other group showing apparently time-related progressive histological signs of recurrent diabetic nephropathy. Consequently, it is possible that genetic factors play an important role in the development of the diabetic nephropathy. At present it has been well demonstrated by Barbosa *et al.* [14] in a randomized study that a good glucose homeostasis can prevent the apparition of GBM thickness and mesangium expansion. Therefore, Reichard *et al.* [15] have demonstrated that a good glycemic control (Hb1Ac between 7 and 7.5) decreases at least of 50% the risk of proteinuria.

It is important to remark that after several years a certain percentage of diabetic transplant recipients develop clinically significant diabetic nephropathy in their transplanted kidney. Recurrence of diabetic nephropathy is reported to occur in up to 50% of diabetic recipients. Hariharan *et al.* [16] reported graft failure due to diabetic nephropathy in 50% of the recipients who developed a diabetic glomerulosclerosis of kidney graft. Graft loss recurred generally in a period comprised between 5 and 10 years after transplantation. In this series the development of allograft diabetic nephropathy was associated with a high rate of graft failure.

Transplanted pancreas exerts a protective effect against diabetic nephropathy in kidney grafts

Transplantation of allogeneic pancreatic beta cells, either vascularized allograft or as components of dispersed islets, remains the only reliable means of achieving sustained euglycemia in patients with type I diabetes.

A technically successful pancreas transplantation results in normal or near-normal fasting plasma glucose levels, glucose tolerance tests and levels of HbA1c. Bohman *et al.* [17] in 1985 and Wilckzek *et al.* [12] in 1995 showed that a pancreatic allograft prevents the development of recurrent diabetic nephropathy in a simultaneously transplanted kidney. Bilous *et al.* [18] in 1989 showed that successful pancreas transplantation is associated with significantly less severe diabetic glomerulopathy in kidney previously transplanted into diabetic patients. Despite the results of these studies, confirming the hypothesis that pancreas transplantation correcting the abnormal metabolic milieu prevents further complications of diabetes has proved difficult. Indeed, the majority of the studies have examined patients for relatively brief periods achieving contrasting results. Consequently, our group [19] decided to analyze renal function and structure in simultaneous pancreas-kidney recipients with functioning kidney and pancreas *versus* recipients who have lost their pancreas graft and present functioning kidney graft alone. Ten years after transplantation the recipients who have lost their pancreas showed an increase in albumin urinary excretion, a progressive thickening of glomerular and tubular basement membrane and an expansion of glomerular and mesangial volume. Although the structural alterations were shown in the group with functioning kidney alone, all recipients from both groups presented normal serum creatinine at the study time. These findings demonstrated that glomerular lesions precede the clinical signs of the diabetic nephropathy as well as the protective effect of pancreas transplantation against the recurrence of the diabetic nephropathy in kidney grafts.

Recent studies [20] have also demonstrated that long-term survival in diabetic patients undergoing simultaneous pancreas-kidney transplantation is better than in diabetic patients receiving kidney transplant alone.

In addition, it has been shown [21] reversal of lesions of diabetic nephropathy after pancreas transplantation in patients with type I diabetes who did not receive kidney allograft. It is very interesting that reversal requires more than 5 years of normoglycemia.

All these data suggest that, despite the initial increase in hospitalization time and complications, pancreas transplantation has progressed to the point where the long-term benefits outweigh the risks.

Metabolic effects of restoring total or partial beta cell function after islet allotransplantation

Successful intraportal islet transplantation normalizes glucose metabolism in type I diabetic patients and prevents the development of the chronic complications associated with the disease [22]. The major factors limiting the large-scale application of islet graft in diabetic patients receiving chronic immunosuppression for a kidney graft are the low percentage of patients reaching insulin independence. The majority of patients achieve only partial function and a reduction of the pretransplant insulin requirement. Long-term results in patients with partial graft function showed that restoring partial function of the secretory capacity of beta cells can lead to the normalization of protein and lipid metabolism with the persistence of mild alteration of glucose homeostasis [23]. Recent data in rodents have suggested a biological activity for the C-peptide, which plays an important role in the delay and prevention of microvascular complications of diabetes. Consequently, a good metabolic control of type I diabetes can be also achieved with a partially functioning pancreatic islet graft.

Finally, in light of the recent data showing that pancreas and islet transplantation can influence the evolution of the lesions of diabetic nephropathy, these procedures have emerged as an important option for the management of patients with insulin-dependent diabetes mellitus and diabetic nephropathy.

References

1. Osterby R. The number of glomerular cells and substructures in early juvenile diabetes. *Acta Path Microbiol Scand* 1972; A80: 785-800.
2. Steffes MW, Osterby R, Chavers B, Mauer M. Mesangial expansion as a central mechanism for loss of kidney function in diabetic patients. *Diabetes* 1989; 38: 1077-81.
3. Mauer SM, Steffes MW, Sutherland DER, Brown DM, Goetz FC. Structural-functional relationships in diabetic nephropathy. *J Clin Invest* 1984; 74: 1143-55.
4. Osterby R, Parving HH, Nyberg G, Hommel E, Jorgensen HE, Lokkegaard H, Svalander C. A strong correlation between glomerular filtration rate and filtration surface in diabetic nephropathy. *Diabetologia* 1983; 31: 265-70.
5. Bilous RW. Can we prevent or delay diabetic nephropathy? *J R Coll Physicians Lond* 1997; 31: 22-7.
6. Rasch R. Prevention of diabetic nephropathy in streptozotocin diabetic rats by insulin treatment: the mesangial regions. *Diabetologia* 1979; 17: 243-8.
7. DCCT Research Group. The effect of intensive treatment of diabetes on the development and progression of long-term complications in insulin-dependent diabetes mellitus. *N Engl J Med* 1993; 329: 977-86.
8. Steffes MW. Glomerular lesions of diabetes mellitus: preventable and reversible. *Nephrol Dial Transplant* 1999; 14: 19-21.

9. Mauer SM, Barbosa J, Vernier RL, Kjellstrand CM, Buselmeier TJ, Simmons RL, Najarian JS, Goetz FC. Development of diabetic vascular lesions in normal kidneys transplanted into patients with diabetes mellitus. *N Engl J Med* 1976; 295: 916-20.
10. Osterby R, Nyberg G, Hedman L, Karlberg I, Persson H, Svalander C. Kidney transplantation in type I (insulin-dependent) diabetic patients. *Diabetologia* 1991; 34: 668-74.
11. Mauer SM, Steffes MW, Connett J, Najarian JS, Sutherland DER, Barbosa J. The development of lesions in the glomerular basement membrane and mesangium after transplantation of normal kidneys to diabetic patients. *Diabetes* 1983; 32: 948-52.
12. Wilckzek HE, Jaremko G, Tyden G, Groth CG. Evolution of diabetic nephropathy in kidney grafts. Evidence that a simultaneously transplanted pancreas exerts a protective effect. *Transplantation* 1995; 59: 51-7.
13. Mauer SM, Goetz FC, McHugh LE, Sutherland DER, Barbosa J, Najarian JS, Steffes MW. Long-term study of normal kidneys transplanted into diabetic patients with type I diabetes. *Diabetes* 1989; 38: 516-23.
14. Barbosa J, Steffes MW, Sutherland DER, Connett JE, Rako KV, Mauer SM. Effect of glycemic control on early diabetic renal lesions. *JAMA* 1994; 272: 600-6.
15. Reichard P, Nilsson BY, Rosenquist U. The effect of long-term intensified insulin treatment on the devepment of microvascular complication of diabetes mellitus. *N Engl J Med* 1993; 329: 977-86.
16. Hariharan S, Smith RD, Viero R, First MR. Diabetic nephropathy after renal transplantation. Clinical and pathological features. *Transplantation* 1996; 62: 632-5.
17. Bohman SO, Tyden G, Wilczek H, Lundgren G, Jaremko G, Gunnarsson R, Ostman J, Groth CG. Prevention of kidney graft diabetic nephropathy by pancreas transplantation in man. *Diabetes* 1985; 34: 306-8.
18. Bilous RW, Mauer SM, Sutherland DER, Najarian JS, Goetz FC, Steffes MW. The effects of pancreas transplantation on the glomerular structure on renal allografts in patients with insulin-dependent diabetes. *N Engl J Med* 1989; 321: 80-5.
19. Lefrancois N, Hadjaissa A, Petruzzo P, Da Silva M, Martin X, Dubernard JM, Touraine JL. Impact of pancreas function on long-term renal function in simultaneous pancreas-kidney transplantation. *Transplant Proc* 2000; 32: 2774-5.
20. Smets YFC, Westendorp RGJ, van der Pijl JW, de Charro FT, Ringers J, de Fijter JW, Lemkes HHPJ. Effect of simultaneous pancreas-kidney transplantation on mortality of patients with type-1 diabetes mellitus and stage renal disease. *Lancet* 1999; 353: 1915-9.
21. Fioretto P, Steffes MW, Sutherland DER, Goetz CG, Mauer M. Reversal of lesions of diabetic nephropathy after pancreas transplantation. *N Engl J Med* 1998; 339: 69-75.
22. Masetti M, Inverardi L, Ranuncoli A, Iaria G, Lupo F, Vizzardelli C, Kenyon NS, Alejandro R, Ricordi C. Current indications and limits of pancreatic islet transplantation in diabetic nephropathy. *J Nephrol* 1997; 10: 245-52.
23. Luzi L, Perseghin G, Brendel MD, Terruzzi I, Battezzati A, Eckhard M, Brandhorst D, Brandhorst H, Friemann S, Socci C, Di Carlo V, Sereni LP, Benedini S, Secchi A, Pozza G, Bretzel RG. Metabolic effects of restoring partial beta cell function after islet alltransplantation in type-1 diabetic patients. *Diabetes* 2001; 50: 277-82.

Thrombotic complications

Thrombotic complications play an important role in early graft losses in lupus patients, especially when antiphospholipid antibodies (APAs) are present. APAs are directed against the β2-glycoprotein I rather than the phospholipid itself. They prolong phospholipid-dependent coagulation *in vitro*, but are associated with thrombosis *in vivo*. APAs have been reported to be present in 30-44% of patients with SLE. After transplantation, renal-artery or vein thrombosis has also been reported in lupus patients, and according to one report, renal artery thrombosis was responsible for 6% of graft losses when APAs were present. The role of APAs was stressed by Radhakrishman [22]. In SLE patients, these authors reported four thrombotic events in five patients who were APA positive, *vs* none in five APA-negative patients. However, these events were not associated with graft loss or death. In the absence of a controlled prospective trial, patients with APA and a history of recurrent thrombosis who undergo transplantation should be treated with effective anticoagulation, both during and after transplantation.

Immunosuppressive treatment

To date, no study has dealt either with the effects of new immunosuppressive drugs on short- and long-term survival, or with the incidence of recurrent nephritis. Among new treatment, mycophenolate mofetil (MMF) and co-stimulation inhibitors are promising.

MMF was found to be effective in the prevention of progressive nephritis in a murine model of SLE [23]. In humans, both encouraging results and less successful uncontrolled experience have been reported. A controlled trial is urgently needed. The effects of antibodies against the co-stimulatory molecules CD154 and B7 have also been evaluated in animal models of renal transplantation and lupus nephritis, and these antibodies will probably be used in the future.

Conclusion

Renal transplantation is a good alternative for management of SLE patients with ESRD. However, data permitting comparison of the effects of renal transplantation and dialysis are lacking. Lupus patients carry a higher risk of thrombosis events and perhaps of immunological failure The rate of clinical recurrent nephritis is low. For us and according to other reports, the SLE biological activity before transplantation does not predict an eventual recurrence, and must not be a criterion for delaying renal transplantation.

Because many patients have received immunosuppressive drugs before transplantation, special attention should be paid to the choice of anti-infectious strategy. In the long term, neoplastic complications may also be more frequent in ESRD patients with SLE. Assessment of the thrombotic risk before transplantation is also important. The presence of APAs indicates the need for active anticoagulation.

References

1. Advisory Committee to the Renal Transplant Registry. Renal transplantation in congenital and metabolic diseases: a report from ASC/NIH renal transplant registry. *JAMA* 1975; 232: 148-53.
2. Cheigh JS, Kim H, Stenzel KH, Tapia L, Sullivan JF, Studenbord W, Riggio RR, Rubin AL. Systemic lupus erythematosus in patients end-stage renal disease: long term follow-up on the prognosis of patients and the evolution of lupus activity. *Am J Kidney Dis* 1990; 16: 189-95.
3. Bumgardner GL, Mauer SM, Payne W, Dunn DL, Sutherland DER, Fryd DS, Ascher NL, Simmons RL, Najarian JS. Single center 1-15 year results of renal transplantation in patients with systemic lupus erythematosus. *Transplantation* 1988; 46: 703-9.
4. Krishnan G, Thacker L, Angstadt JD, Capelli JP. Multicenter analysis of renal allograft suvival in lupus patients. *Transplant Proc* 1991; 23: 1755-6.
5. Hariharan S, Schroeder TJ, Carey MA, First MR. Renal transplantation in patients with systemic lupus erythematosus. *Clin Transplant* 1992; 6: 345-9.
6. Sumrani N, Miles AM, Delaney V, Daskalakis P, Markell M, Hong JH. Renal transplantation in cyclosporine-treated patients with end-stage lupus nephropathy. *Transplant Proc* 1992; 24: 1785-7.
7. Lochhead K, Pirsch J, D'Alessandro A, Knechtle S, Kalayoglu M, Sollinger H, Belzer F. Risk factors for renal allograft loss in patients with systemic lupus erythematosus. *Kidney Int* 1996; 49: 515-7.
8. Cats S, Galton J. Effect of original disease in kidney transplant outcome. In: Terasaki PI, ed. *Clinical transplants*. Los Angeles, UCLA Tissue Typing Laboratory, 1985: 111-21.
9. Nyberg G, Karlberg I, Svalander C, Hedman L, Blohme I. Renal transplantation in patients with systemic lupus erythematosus. Increased risk of early graft loss. *Scand J Urol Nephro* 1990; 24: 307-13.
10. Cattran DC, April M. Renal transplantation in systemic lupus erythematosus. *Ann Intern Med* 1991; 114: 991.
11. Grimbert P, Frappier J, Bedrossian J, et al. for The Groupe Cooperatif de Transplantation d'Ile de France. Long-term outcome of kinase transplantation in patients with systemic lupus erythematosus. *Transplantation* 1998; 66: 1000-3.
12. Ward MM. Outomes of renal transplantation among patients with end-stage renal disease caused by lupus nephritis. *Kidney Int* 2000; 57: 2136-43.
13. Roth D, Milgrom M, Esquenazi V, Strauss J, Zilleruelo G, Miller J. Renal transplantation in systemic lupus erythematosus. *Am J Nephrol* 1987; 7: 367-74.
14. Goss JA, Cole BR, Jendrisak MD, McCullough CS, So SKS, Windus DW, Hanto DW. Renal transplantation for systemic lupus erythematosus and recurrent lupus nephritis. *Transplantation* 1991; 52: 805-10.
15. Kumano K, Sakai T, Mashimo S, Endo T, Koshiba K, Elises JS, Iitaka K. A case of recurrent lupus nephritis after transplant. *Clin Nephrol* 1987; 27: 94-8.
16. Fernandez JA, Milgrom M, Burke GW, Miller J, Roth D. Recurrence of lupus nephritis in a renal allograft with histologic transformation of the lesion. *Transplantation* 1990; 50: 1056-8.
17. Amend WJC, Vicenti F, Feduska NJ, Salvatierra O, Johnston WH, Jackson J, Tilnet N, Burwell EL. Recurrent systemic lupus erythematosus involving renal allografts. *Ann Intern Med* 1981; 94: 444-8.
18. Sohmiya S, Morozumi K, Yoshida A. A case of recurrent lupus nephritis after renal transplantation immunosuppressed with cyclosporine. *Jap J Transplant* 1986; 21: 18-20.
19. Moorthy V, Zimmerman SW, Mejla G, Sollinger HW, Belzer FO. Recurrent lupus nephritis after renal transplantation. *Kidney Int* 1987; 31: 464.
20. Stone JH, Millward CL, Olson JL, Amend WJ. Frequency of recurrent lupus nephritis among ninety-seven renal transplant patients during the cyclosporine era. *Arthritis Rheum* 1998; 41: 678-86.
21. Nyberg G, Blohme I, Persson H, Olausson M, Svalander C. Recurrence of systemic lupus erythematosus in transplanted kidneys: a follow-up transplant biopsy study. *Nephrol Dial Transplant* 1992; 7: 1116-23.
22. Radhakrishnan J, Williams GS, Appel GB, Cohen DJ. Renal transplantation in anticardiolipin antibois-positive lupus erythematosus patients. *Am J Kidney Dis* 1994; 23: 286-9.
23. Van Bruggen MC, Walgreen B, Rijke TP, Verden JH. Attenuation of murine lupus nephritis by mycophenolate mofetil. *J Am Soc Nephrol* 1998; 9: 1407-15.

Conservative treatment

Therapy should start as early as possible, but is frequently delayed, as diagnosis of PH 1 is often only made many years after the first symptoms have occurred [13, 14]. Conservative treatment includes a high daily fluid intake (> 2-3 L/24 h) to increase the urine volume. Pyridoxine may effectively decrease the endogenous oxalate production [2, 14], since pyridoxal phosphate is a cofactor of AGT. However, only a minority of patients ($\simeq$ 33%) respond to such therapy [14]. In addition the administration of alkali citrate or orthophosphate is necessary to increase the urinary solubility product [15, 16]. Nevertheless, in most patients unresponsive to pyridoxine, recurrent urolithiasis or progressive nephrocalcinosis will still occur leading to kidney damage and ultimately to end stage renal failure [14].

Dialysis

Neither haemodialysis (HD) nor peritoneal dialysis (PD) are able to keep pace with the continuing overproduction of oxalate in PH 1 patients, much less to reduce the body oxalate burden [8, 17]. In fact, the weekly oxalate dialysance of renal replacement therapies (6-9 mmol/week) only equals the endogenous oxalate production of two to three days [17, 18]. Therefore, oxalate is gradually accumulating, and CaOx crystals are, next to the kidney, deposited in other organs, soft tissue, bones and in the retina [2, 5, 14]. The longer the period of dialysis, the worse the prognosis even after a primarily successful transplantation [13, 19]. No form of dialysis is therefore an alternative to transplantation, and even intensive dialysis, *e.g.* the combination of HD and PD or intensified HD, can only be regarded as a bridging procedure for not more than a few months.

Transplantation

Transplantation, be it isolated kidney, isolated liver or combined transplantation, needs to be planned early so as to avoid any dialysis, or at least any long period of dialysis. Which transplantation procedure should be chosen? First, the decision has to take into account the previous clinical course and the urinary excretion parameters under medication. A patient whose urinary oxalate excretion does not decrease with pyridoxine medication and who has recurrent urolithiasis and/or progressive nephrocalcinosis is not a candidate for isolated kidney transplantation, not even from a living related donor [14]. The risk of recurrence is high, as the amount of urinary oxalate excretion will remain unchanged. In addition, an even higher oxalate excretion immediately after transplantation, due to mobilisation of body oxalate stores, may lead to early recurrence and even graft failure *(Figure 1)*. In contrast, this procedure might be considered for pyridoxine responsive cases with near normalisation of urinary oxalate excretion [20] or, perhaps, for elderly patients with a mild clinical form of PH 1.

Isolated kidney transplantation is, however, still recommended in the United States, and a strict post-transplant protocol with aggressive therapy is used to minimise the risk of early recurrence [21, 22]. This concept includes a high fluid intake, the admi-

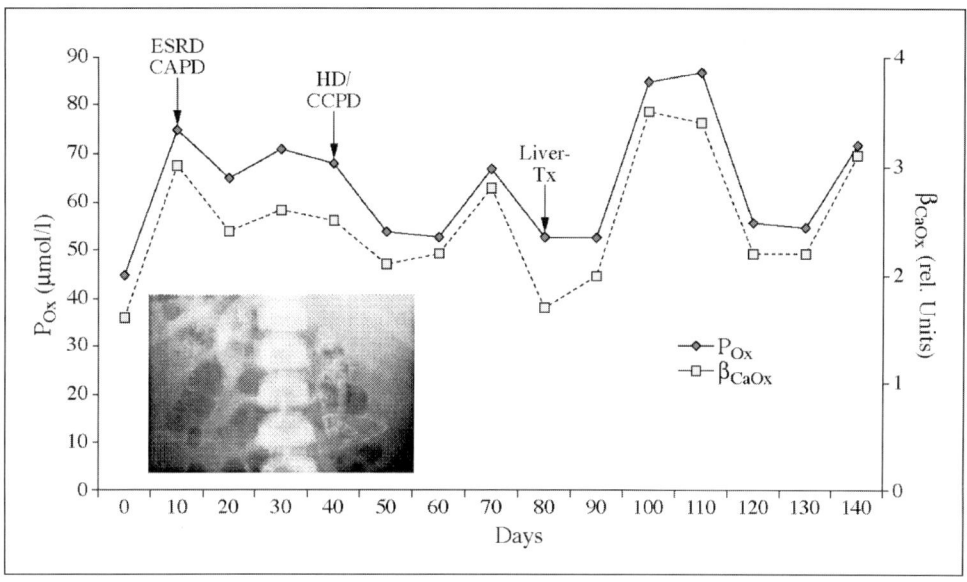

Figure 1. P_{Ox} and $β_{CaOx}$ in a 6 years old girl with PH 1 and systemic oxalosis after an isolated kidney transplant had failed due to immediate recurrence in the graft. P_{Ox} and $β_{CaOx}$ remained strongly elevated over time, although a combination of HD (6 x 3.5 h per week) and PD treatment was performed. A first liver transplantat functioned only poorly, and the patient died shortly before retransplantation. Abdominal X-ray showed severe nephrocalcinosis in the native kidneys.

nistration of pyridoxine (even in primarily unresponsive patients) and of citrate or orthophosphate, and, in addition, post-transplant haemodialysis with the aim to reduce the body oxalate burden [22]. The overall transplant survival seems acceptable with 51% graft survival after 6 years and 35% at 10 years [22]. In contrast, previous experiences in Europe clearly showed that transplant survival is much worse in patients with isolated kidney transplantation, as compared to combined liver-kidney transplantation [13, 19]. Three year transplant survival rates were only 23% for living donors and 17% for cadaveric kidneys [23].

Isolated (pre-emptive) liver Tx has been performed in a few centres [24]. The rationale is to cure the enzyme defect before renal insufficiency occurs, so that no kidney graft will ultimately be required [25, 26]. Indeed, liver transplantation is at present the only form of gene therapy available in PH 1. The crux, however, is the optimal timing, which is extremely difficult as primary hyperoxaluria is a very heterogeneous disease with an unpredictable course [24-27]. GFR should certainly not be less than 40 ml/min, but rather exceed 50 ml/min [26, 27]. With such a GFR the P_{Ox} would remain < 30 μmol/l, hence the plasma would not become supersaturated with respect to calcium-oxalate [10, 12].

More than a dozen patients with PH I have been treated this way with reasonable results [25, 26]. If the GFR is < 40 ml/min before liver transplantation, the risk of a rapid further decline necessitating secondary kidney transplantation is high [26]. The benefits of this procedure correlate therefore strongly with residual kidney function. On the other hand, patients with maintained renal function may remain stable and may not require any transplantation procedure at all for many years *(Figure 2)*.

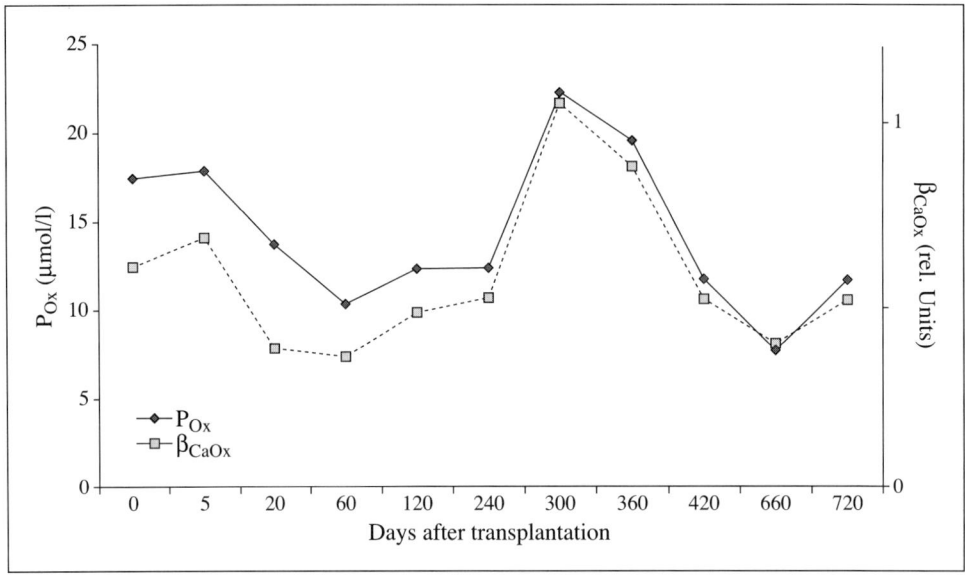

Figure 2. P_{Ox} and β_{CaOx} remained moderately elevated in a 13 years old boy with PH I after preemptive liver-transplantation. His GFR remained stable over time (64 ml/min x 1.73 m^2).

Liver transplantation in PH 1 is a major procedure, as it is necessary to remove the otherwise healthy liver to cure the metabolic defect. Auxiliary liver transplantation has no place, as overproduction of oxalate by the patient's own liver would persist [2, 26]. If liver function is satisfactory, oxalate production returns to normal and no further calcium-oxalate deposition takes place [26]. However, the use of calcineurin inhibitors may further compromise residual renal function.

Combined liver-kidney transplantation is the recommended strategy in Europe [13, 19], as by this procedure both the enzyme defect is cured and renal function is restored. Although the endogenous oxalate production is immediately normalised, both P_{Ox} and β_{PcaOx}, and particularly the hyperoxaluria, will persist for months or even years, depending on the extent of generalised CaOx deposits that are mobilised (*Figure 3*, [6, 8]). This demonstrates again that PH 1 patients have extremely high body CaOx stores [28]. In contrast, the increased plasma oxalate levels in non-PH patients are normalised within 3 weeks after transplantation [8]. Therefore, the earlier the transplantation, the less the body oxalate burden and the lower the risk of recurrent oxalate deposition in the transplanted kidney.

Aggressive post-transplant measures are needed because the risk of recurrent oxalate deposits for any patient is greatest immediately after transplantation [20]. While intensive dialysis until transplantation, and during (transient) renal graft dysfunction, is essential, additional haemodialysis or haemofiltration adds very little to overall oxalate removal in well functioning grafts. Young patients with the infantile form of oxalosis with severe nephrocalcinosis may require a constant and large fluid intake by gastrostomy for many months (*Figure 3*, [29]).

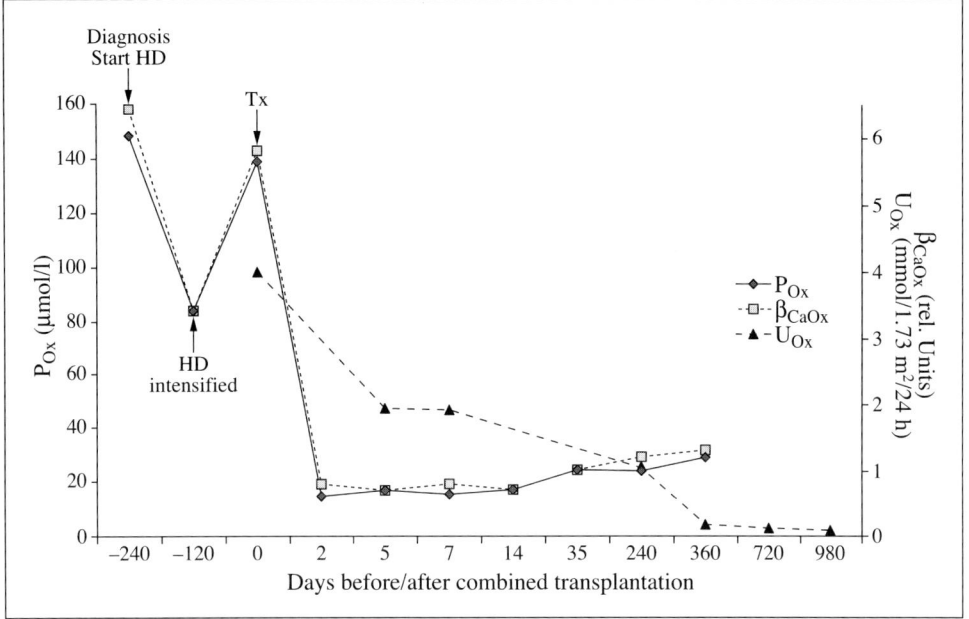

Figure 3. Boy with end stage renal failure due to infantile oxalosis diagnosed at 3 months and treated by haemodialysis until successful combined-liver kidney transplantation at the age of 15 months. Stable transplant function (GFR 80 ml/min x 1.73 m^2) 4 years later. Post-transplant treatment included an extreme fluid intake primarily using a gastrostomy tube. Urinary oxalate excretion slowly decreased from 4 mmol/1.73 m^2/24 h directly after transplantation to 1.1 mmol/1.73 m^2/24 h after 12 months. Normal levels were reached 2 years after transplantation.

An alternative for a patient who has already developed severe generalised oxalosis is to transplant first the liver, then to reduce the body oxalate burden *via* aggressive haemodialysis, and in a second stage to perform kidney transplantion [30]. By this way the risk of recurrent oxalate deposition is reduced at the price of two consecutive transplants from different donors.

According to the European Oxalosis Registry, more than 100 combined liver/kidney transplantations have been reported in Europe with an 80% patient survival at 5 years with liver graft survival of 71% [5, 19]. Notably, renal function has remained stable with creatinine clearances between 40 and 60 ml/min after 5 years [19].

Conclusion

Primary hyperoxaluria type 1 is a very heterogeneous disease, with rapid disease progression into renal failure in many patients. Diagnosis needs to be made early, but this is rarely achieved; accordingly, medical treatment is frequently delayed. The risk of developing systemic oxalosis is high in patients with PH 1, and the more oxalate accumulates, the lower is the chance of a good outcome, even after successful transplantation. Early combined liver-kidney transplantation or, exceptionally, pre-emptive liver transplantation, is at present the best option to avoid progressive systemic oxalosis.

Recurrence of membranoproliferative glomerulonephritis after renal transplantation

Rémi Cahen

Service de Néphrologie, Centre Hospitalier Lyon Sud, Pierre-Bénite, France

Recurrent diseases in the kidney transplant are now recognized more frequently as graft survival continues to improve due to better management of acute rejection. However, assessing the diagnosis of recurrent or *de novo* glomerulonephritis requires an accurate diagnosis of the histopathological lesions in the transplanted kidney and knowledge that the transplanted kidney had a normal histology at the time of implantation. Many patients entering an end-stage renal failure treatment program do not have a biopsy undertaken and furthermore a number of transplanted patients with urinary abnormalities and/or poor renal function similarly do not have a biopsy performed. Finally, a recurrent glomerulonephritis can be clinically silent and detected only by a routine transplant biopsy. All these factors would lead to underestimate the prevalence of recurrent glomerulonephritis.

Membranoproliferative glomerulonephritis (MPGN), also called mesangiocapillary glomerulonephritis, is an immune complex-mediated glomerulonephritis characterized by diffuse mesangial cell proliferation and matrix expansion and thickening of the capillary wall. There has been a decline in the incidence of MPGN over the past two decades from 10-20% to 2-6% of primary glomerulonephritides in North America and Europe [1]. This is best explained by a change in environmental factors, particularly infectious organisms [1]. MPGN can be primary (idiopathic) or secondary (associated diseases including cryoglobulinemia and viral infections). MPGN is classified as type I when the immune deposits are in the subendothelial space and in the mesangium, type II when dense deposits are present within the glomerular basement membrane (GBM) and type III when immune deposits are diffusely present in the subendothelium, within the GBM and in the subepithelial space. Type I MPGN is by far the most frequent. In this paper, we will consider the recurrence of the three types of MPGN and the association of MPGN with hepatitis C virus (HCV) after renal transplantation.

Type I MPGN

Rate of recurrence

In a recent overview of 179 cases of renal transplantation for type I MPGN from 11 studies published in the literature, the recurrence rate varied from 9% to 53% with a mean of 30% [2]. More recently, Lien *et al.* [3] selected 14 previously published studies, that provided adequate information on the incidence and outcome of recurrence. Sixty one out of a total of 218 patients (28%) developed recurrent type I MPGN. These percentages are similar to the 30% reported in the comprehensive review by Cameron in 1982 [4]. In their personal series of 27 recipients of a first cadaveric graft, Andresdottir *et al.* [2] found a recurrence rate of 33%, but a cumulative incidence of 48% at 4 years after transplantation when patients with graft failure from other causes were censored. The same authors found a 75% recurrence rate in 4 recipients of HLA living related donor (LRD) grafts. The recurrence rate increased up to 80% in recipients of a second cadaver graft who had a recurrence in their first graft [2].

In children, Habib [5] reported a recurrence in 7 out of 10 renal allograft recipients who had a routine biopsy with immunofluorescence (IF) study. When a graft biopsy was performed only when clinically indicated, The North American Pediatric Renal Transplantation Cooperative Study [6] reported a recurrence with graft loss in only one patient out of 14 (7%) transplanted for type I MPGN and Müller *et al.* [7] in a single center study found no recurrence in 3 allografts for type I MPGN with a mean follow-up of 5.3 years.

Histopathology

The reported rate of recurrence may reflect an overestimate of the true incidence because histological distinction between recurrent type I MPGN and allograft glomerulopathy may be difficult [8]. On light microscopy the lesions are very similar. However, glomerular crescents can be seen in type I MPGN, but not in transplant glomerulopathy, while intimal thickening of the arteries and interstitial fibrosis are usually associated with transplant glomerulopathy. These two entities can reliably be distinguished by IF and electron microscopy (EM). In patients with type I MPGN, IF study shows prominent granular deposits in the capillary wall, and to a lesser extent in the mesangium, of C3 with lesser amounts of IgG and IgM. In patients with transplant glomerulopathy, IF shows glomerular IgM deposits. On EM, patients with recurrent MPGN show electron-dense deposits on the subendothelial side of the glomerular basement membrane, while patients with allograft glomerulopathy never show deposits but show widening of the subendothelial space of the capillary wall, which contains electron-lucent material [8].

Clinical presentation and graft outcome

Recurrence may be clinically silent and purely histologic, as reported by Habib *et al.* [5] in 5 out of 7 children with recurrence followed between 2 and 9 years. Recurrence can present as proteinuria and microscopic hematuria, nephrotic syndrome, with or without renal failure. Two of the 7 children (29%) reported by Habib *et al.* [5] had proteinuria and finally lost their graft because of recurrence within 13 months. In one patient, the disease recurred in a second graft. In the study by Andresdottir *et al.* [2], the patients with recurrent type I MPGN presented with proteinuria of more than 1 g/day detected 1.5 to 42 months post transplantation with progression to the nephrotic syndrome in almost all of them. Among the 12 patients with recurrence, 7 (58%) lost their graft due to recurrence [2]. This rate of graft failure is comparable to the 55% reported by Lien *et al.* [3] in 61 patients with recurrent type I MPGN from 14 previously published studies. It is also close to the 66% of graft failure of 18 patients with recurrent or *de novo* MPGN reported by Hariharian *et al.* [9] from the Renal Allograft Disease Registry. The relative risk of graft failure because of recurrent MPGN was 2.37. Patients with MPGN after transplantation had a 5-year graft survival of 32.2%, significantly lower than the 67.6% for patients without recurrence or *de novo* disease [9]. Andresdottir *et al.* [2] found a mean duration of graft survival of 40 months after the appearance of proteinuria. In recipients of HLA identical grafts, it has been shown that recurrent glomerulonephritis is the major cause of graft loss. Up to 50% of surviving patients transplanted for a glomerulonephritis will progress to end-stage renal disease as a result of recurrence of the original disease [10].

Risk factors of recurrence

Gender and age at diagnosis were not associated with the risk of recurrence [2]. Whether the rate of progression of the original disease on native kidneys, the time on dialysis, the interval between first and second transplant are prognostic factors remains to be determined [2, 11]. However, rapidly progressive disease in native kidneys with glomerular crescents may be associated with a similar course in a first transplant [4, 11]. The haplotype HLA B8 DR3 was associated with a higher risk of recurrence in the series of cadaveric transplant recipients studied by Andresdottir *et al.* [2]. No other study has shown an association between HLA alleles and recurrence of type I MPGN. The high recurrence rate (75%) reported by Andresdottir *et al.* [2] in the recipients of an HLA identical LRD graft suggests that the genetic similarities between donor and recipient might increase the risk of recurrence. However, it has not been demonstrated thus far that type I MPGN recurs more likely in LRD grafts as compared to cadaveric donor grafts [2, 11].

There have been conflicting reports on the value of hypocomplementemia as a risk factor of recurrence. Berthoux *et al.* [12] found that patients with recurrence of the original disease had hypocomplementemia after transplantation, while those without recurrence maintained normal levels of complement. However, Mclean *et al.* [13] did not find a clear correlation between hypocomplementemia after transplantation and recurrence. Andresdottir *et al.* [2] showed that recurrence occurred in patients with low as well as normal C3 levels before and after transplantation. It is now agreed that presence and severity of complement abnormalities is not predictive of recurrence [2, 4].

Native nephrectomy has been previously proposed with the aim to prevent recurrent glomerulonephritides after transplantation. However, Odorico *et al.* [14] showed in a retrospective study that the rate of recurrence and graft failure was not significantly influenced by bilateral nephrectomy.

There has been no reported benefit of cyclosporine or the newer immunosuppressive agents on recurrent or *de novo* glomerulonephritis after transplantation [2, 14].

The potential role of viruses has been largely shown by the relationship between HCV infection and MPGN, both in native [15] and transplanted [16] kidneys. Andres-

MPGN associated with HCV infection

Roth et al. [16] in 1995 first reported this association in renal transplant recipients. They described 5 patients from a cohort of 98 HCV-positive renal transplant recipients, who presented a *de novo* MPGN after renal transplantation. All had nephrotic-range proteinuria and HCV RNA in the serum. None of these patients had cryoglobulinemia, but 2 had hypocomplementemia and rhumatoid factor. Circulating complexes were detected in one patient. More recently, Cruzado et al. [27] described 6 HCV-positive patients with nephrotic-range proteinuria, microscopic hematuria and *de novo* MPGN. Low levels of circulating immune complexes and cryoglobulins were noted in all patients, which were type II cryoglobulins (IgMk monoclonal), as it was reported in native kidneys [15]. Hypocomplementemia was detected in all patients. HCV RNA was found in higher concentrations in cryoprecipitate than in serum, suggesting that HCV participated in formation of cryoglobulins. Renal biopsy led to the diagnosis of cryoglobulinemic MPGN.

Brunkhorst et al. [28] described the first case of recurrent type I MPGN 2 years after transplantation in a patient with chronic HCV infection and HCV RNA in the serum. Hammoud et al. [29] showed in a cohort of 399 renal transplant recipients, 117 of whom were HCV-positive, that the proportion of patients that developed a MPGN was higher in HCV-positive (6.8%) than in HCV-negative (2.5%) patients.

Thus, these studies have demonstrated that HCV infection after renal transplantation is associated with *de novo* or recurrent type I MPGN, with or without cryoglobulinemia, despite immunosuppressive therapy. In the same way, HCV-positive liver transplant patients can also develop type II cryobulinemia, proteinuria and MPGN [30].

Many articles describing the recurrence of type I MPGN in renal allograft were published prior to the description of the association between HCV and MPGN. Consequently, some of those reports may have overestimated the recurrence rate of idiopathic type I MPGN.

The treatment has not yet been defined. Alpha-interferon can induce renal dysfunction in transplanted patients [31]. Ribavirin has been reported to be effective in HCV-associated nephrotic syndrome in liver transplant recipients [32]. Cyclophosphamide may be useful in transplanted patients with cryoglobulinemic MPGN [33].

References

1. William DG. Mesangiocapillary glomerulonephritis. In: Davison AM, Cameron JS, Grünfeld JP, Kerr DNS, Ritz E, Wineals CG, eds. *Oxford textbook of clinical nephrology*. Oxford: Oxford University Press, 1998: 591-612.
2. Andresdottir MB, Assmann KJM, Hoitsma AJ, et al. Recurrence of type I membranoproliferative glomerulonephritis after renal transplantation. *Transplantation* 1997; 63: 1628-33.
3. Lien YH, Scott K. Long-term cyclophosphamide treatment for recurrent type I membranoproliferative glomerulonephritis after transplantation. *Am J Kidney Dis* 2000; 35: 539-43.
4. Cameron JS. Glomerulonephritis in renal transplants. *Transplantation* 1982; 34: 237-44.
5. Habib R, Antignac C, Hinglais N, et al. Glomerular lesions in the transplanted kidney in children. *Am J Kidney Dis* 1987; 10: 198-207.

6. Alexander SR, Arbus GS, Butt KMH, et al.. The 1989 Report of the North American Pediatric Renal Transplant Cooperative Study. *Pediatr Nephrol* 1990; 4: 542-53.
7. Müller T, Sikora P, Offner G, et al. Recurrence of renal disease after kidney transplantation in children: 24 years of experience in a single center. *Clin Nephrol* 1998; 49: 82-90.
8. Andresdottir MB, Assmann KJM, Koene RAP, et al. Immunohistological and ultrastructural differences between recurrent type I membranoproliferative glomerulonephritis and chronic transplant glomerulopathy. *Am J Kidney Dis* 1998; 32: 582-8.
9. Hariharan S, Adams MB, Brennan DC, et al. Recurrent et *de novo* glomerular disease after renal transplantation. *Transplantation* 1999; 68: 635-41.
10. Andresdottir MB, Hoitsma AJ, Assmann KJM, et al. The impact of recurrent glomerulonephritis on graft survival in recipients of human histocompatibility leucocyte antigen-identical living related donor grafts. *Transplantation* 1999; 68: 623-7.
11. Glicklich D, Matas AJ, Sablay LB, et al. Recurrent membranoproliferative glomerulonephritis type I in successive renal transplants. *Am J Nephrol* 1987; 7: 143-9.
12. Berthoux FC, Ducret F, Colon S, et al. Renal transplantation in mesangioproliferative glomerulonephritis: relation between the high frequency of recurrent glomerulonephritis and hypocomplementemia. *Kidney Int* 1975; 7: S 323-7.
13. Mclean RH, Geiger H, Burke B, et al. Recurrence of membranoproliferative glomerulonephritis following kidney transplantation: serum complement component study. *Am J Med* 1976; 60: 60-72.
14. Odorico JS, Knechtle SJ, Rayhill SC, et al. The influence of native nephrectomy on the incidence of recurrent disease following renal transplantation for primary glomerulonephritis. *Transplantation* 1996; 61: 228-34.
15. Johnson RH, Gretch DR, Yamabe H, et al. Membranoproliferative glomerulonephritis associated with hepatitis C virus infection. *N Engl J Med* 1993; 328: 465-70.
16. Roth D, Cirocco R, Zucker K, et al. De novo membranoproliferative glomerulonephritis in hepatitis C virus-infected renal allograft recipients. *Transplantation* 1995; 59: 1676-82.
17. Andresdottir MB, Assmann KJM, Hilbrands LB, et al. Primary Epstein-Barr virus infection and recurrent type I membranoproliferative glomerulonephritis after renal transplantation. *Nephrol Dial Transplant* 2000; 15: 1235-7.
18. Andresdottir MB, Assmann KJM, Hilbrands LB, et al. Type I membranoproliferative glomerulonephritis in a renal allograft: a recurrence induced by a cytomegalovirus infection? *Am J Kidney Dis* 2000; 35: E6.
19. Muczinski KA. Plasmapheresis maintained renal function in an allograft with recurrent membranoproliferative glomerulonephritis type I. *Am J Nephrol* 1995; 15: 446-9.
20. Saxena R, Frankel WL, Sedmak DD, et al. Recurrent type I membranoproliferative glomerulonephritis in a renal allograft: successful treatment with plasmapheresis. *Am J Kidney Dis* 2000; 35: 749-52.
21. Cahen R, Trolliet P, Dijoud F, et al. Severe recurrence of type I membranoproliferative glomerulonephritis after transplantation: remission on steroids and cyclophosphamide. *Transpl Proc* 1995; 27: 1746-7.
22. Kotanko P, Pusey CD, Levy J. Recurrent glomerulonephritis following renal transplantation. *Transplantation* 1997; 63: 1045-52.
23. Andresdottir MB, Assmann KJM, Hoitsma AJ, et al. Renal transplantation in patients with dense deposits disease: morphological characteristics of recurrent disease and clinical outcome. *Nephrol Dial Transplant* 1999; 14: 1723-31.
24. Eddy A, Sibley R, Mauer SM, et al. Renal allograft failure due to recurrent dense intramembranous deposits disease. *Clin Nephrol* 1984; 21: 305-13.
25. Oberkircher OR, Enama M, West JC, et al. Regression of recurrent membranoproliferative glomerulonephritis type II in a transplanted kidney after plasmapheresis therapy. *Transpl Proc* 1988; 20 (Suppl. 1): 418-23.
26. Morales JM, Martinez MA, Munoz de Bustillo E, et al. Recurrent type III membrano-proliferative glomerulonephritis after kidney transplantation. *Transplantation* 1997; 63: 1186-8.
27. Cruzado JM, Gil-Vernet S, Ercilla G, et al. Hepatitis C virus-associated membrano-proliferative glomerulonephritis in renal allografts. *J Am Soc Nephrol* 1996; 7: 2469-75.
28. Brunkhorst R, Kliem V, Koch KM. Recurrence of membranoproliferative glomerulo-nephritis after renal transplantation in a patient with chronic hepatitis C. *Nephron* 1996; 72: 465-7.
29. Hammoud H, Haem J, Laurent B, et al. Glomerular disease during HCV infection in renal transplantation. *Nephrol Dial Transplant* 1996; 11 (Suppl. 4): 54-5.

30. Kendrick EA, Mcvicar JP, Kowdley KV, *et al.* Renal disease in hepatitis C-positive liver transplant recipients. *Transplantation* 1997; 63: 1287-93.
31. Rostaing L, Izopet J, Baron E, *et al.* Treatment of chronic hepatitis C with recombinant interferon alpha in kidney transplant recipients. *Transplantation* 1995; 59: 1426-31.
32. Pham HG, Féray C, Samuel D, *et al.* Effects of ribavirin on hepatitis C-associated nephrotic syndrome in four liver transplant recipients. *Kidney Int* 1998; 54: 1311-9.
33. Quigg RJ, Brathwaite M, Gardner DF, *et al.* Successful cyclophosphamide treatment of cryoglobulinemic membranoproliferative glomerulonephritis associated with hepatitis C infection. *Am J Kidney Dis* 1995; 25: 798-800.

Recurrent membranous nephropathy after kidney transplantation

Claire Pouteil-Noble

Transplantation and Nephrology Unit, Centre Hospitalier Lyon-Sud, Pierre-Bénite, France and UFR Lyon-Sud, Université Claude-Bernard

The occurrence of recurrent glomerulopathies has been recognized for over 30 years. All forms of glomerulonephritis can recur following transplantation. The definition of recurrent membranous nephropathy (MN) requires to know precisely the histological diagnosis on the native kidneys.

Membranous nephropathy in the kidney allograft may occur also as a *de novo* MN which would be more frequent than recurrent MN and also theorically as a transmitted MN by the graft.

The first reported case of recurrent membranous nephropathy (MN) was published in 1975 by Crosson [1] and then many isolated cases [2-17] and retrospective series have been reported [18-25]. Only two combined series [23, 26] allowed to estimate the incidence of recurrent MN after kidney transplantation.

The strongest evidence that recurrence do exist comes from the high incidence of MN in the graft in patients with primary MN – that is increased at least three times – compared to that in patients with other causes of renal failure [27].

It is probable that as graft failures from death and rejection decline, the incidence of graft failures from recurrent disease will increase. Among a large cohort of 4,913 subjects with 22% of patients receiving living-related donor transplants, in the Renal Allograft Disease Registry, the incidence of recurrent and *de novo* disease was 3.4% over a mean follow-up period of 5.4 years. MN represented 9.6% of the recurrent glomerulonephritis after focal and segmental glomerulosclerosis (34.1%), IgA nephropathy (13.2%), diabetes (11.4%), membrano-proliferative glomerulonephritis (MPGN) (10.8%) [28]. In children, recurrence of the original disease has been responsible for over 6% of index graft failures and 12% of second graft failures in North America [29].

Prevalence and incidence of recurrent membranous nephropathy

The MN in the native kidney is a rare cause of transplantation. In our experience in 1,614 kidney transplant recipients, MN was the cause of end-stage renal disease in 1.17% (19 cases) and constituted 5.72% of the histologically proven cases of glomerulonephritis [23]. In the Australian and New Zealand dialysis and transplant registry

MN accounts for about 4% of glomerulonephritides causing renal failure [27]. In O'Meara study, the prevalence of MN among the patients with ESRD with histological diagnosis of glomerulonephritis was 6.4% [21]. In Odorico study [25], in 364 patients transplanted with a diagnosis of glomerulonephritis, the prevalence of MN was 17.58%.

This rate may be underestimated since MN is a condition of middle-aged and older patients who may be not offered transplantation. MN is associated with malignancy and such patients may be not candidates for transplantation. However, the MRC glomerulonephritis registry reported only 3.4% of MN associated with neoplasia [30].

The MN recurrence rate after transplantation varies from 4% [19] to 57% [18], with an average of 20% in the largest series [25] *(Table I)*. The time-related probability of recurrence has been estimated from 2 combined series [26] and is of 29% at 3 years with a plateau up to 10 years. In our serie, the rate of recurrence was 26.3% (5/19) [23] and in the University of Louvain, it was of 25% (3/12) [26].

Table I. Prevalence of recurrent membranous nephropathy after kidney transplantation in published series (case reports are excluded)

Authors	Study period	Nb of Tx	Nb of MN	Nb of recurrence	Rate of recurrence
Morzycka et al. [18]	1965-1977	350	7 (2%)	4	57%
Berger et al. [19]	1974-1981	936	25 (2.6%)	1	4%
First et al. [10]	1967-1984	693	NA	3	NA
Honkanen et al. [11]	1964-1982	1 282	NA	1	NA
Montagnino et al. [20]	1969-1983	442	9 (2%)	3	33%
O'Meara et al. [21]	1974-1987	737	10 (1.3%)	1	10%
Schwarz et al. [22]	1970-1988	700	10 (1.4%)	1	10%
Robles et al. [15]	1976-1988	427	NA	3	NA
Lustig et al. [56]	1980-1990	725	11 (1.5%)	4	36%
Couchoud et al. [23]	1980-1993	1,614	19 (1.17%)	5	26%
Marcen et al. [24]	1979-1994	509	6 (1.17%)	3	50%
Odorico et al. [25]	1967-1994	364	64 (17.58%)	13	20.31%
Cosyns et al. [26]	1978-1990	NA	12	3	25%

The variation of the rate of recurrence in the literature is explained by the difference in selection criteria of the patients, by the duration of the follow-up, by the variation of the indication of kidney graft biopsy after transplantation. In our two combined series [26], the selection criteria of included patients were strict: they were selected to have an unquestionable MN before transplantation with morphological evidence of MN in the native kidneys [31]; indications for graft biopsy were homogeneous: persistent proteinuria over 0.2 g/24 hours, impairment of renal function. However, the rate of recurrent MN may be underestimated since MN recurrence may be present without overt proteinuria [32]. Moreover, the true incidence of recurrent MN may be complicated by the occurrence of *de novo* MN in the graft.

Recurrent and *de novo* MN cannot be differentiated on morphological characteristics. In both types, diffuse spikes on the outer surface of the glomerular basement membrane were observed by light microscopy and diffuse epimembranous deposits of IgG along the glomerular basement membrane were visible by immunofluorescent microscopy. Subepithelial electron-dense deposits were observed in the specimens examined by electron microscopy. However *de novo* MN is usually associated with tubulo-interstitial and vascular damage related to chronic rejection.

MN was idiopathic in most of the cases in native kidneys.

In children, MN is a rare cause of ESRF and Broyer report 11 cases of transplantation for MN, and no case of recurrence [33]. In a serie of recurrent disease after kidney transplantation, no case of recurrent MN has been described in the 3 children whose original disease was a MN [34].

Clinical presentation of recurrent membranous nephropathy

The time between MN recurrence and transplantation ranges from 1 week to 148 months in the reported cases, with a mean time of 10 months, while the mean time of *de novo* MN is about 21 months (4 months to 6 years) [26, 30]. In recurrent MN, proteinuria and nephrotic syndrome develop more rapidly than in *de novo* MN and 58% of them occur within 6 months after transplantation [35].

Risk factors for recurrence of membranous nephropathy

Recipient characteristics before transplantation

Several recipient characteristics before or at the time transplantation have been analysed to identify risk factors associated with MN recurrence [23, 26].

It has been suggested that a short evolution of the original disease in native kidneys was associated with an increased risk of recurrence [12]. In the combined series of 30 patients, we did not find any significant difference in the duration of the original disease: 9 years [3-18] in patients with recurrence *versus* 6 years (< 1-22) in patients without recurrence [26]. Thus, duration of MN did not seem to be a predictive factor for MN recurrence.

A prolonged time on hemodialysis (HD) does not prevent recurrence of MN, as it has been suggested by the non-significant difference in the time spent on HD between patients with and without recurrence: 33 months *vs* 29 months respectively [26].

The number of transfusions received before transplantation and the geographic origin were not significantly different in patients with or without recurrence in our study [23].

MN is more severe in male in native kidneys and it is suggested that male patients could have an increased incidence of recurrence [27]. However in our experience, recurrence was not more frequent or severe in male recipients [23].

The immunosuppressive therapy given before dialysis during the course of MN in native kidneys was not associated with a decreased incidence of MN recurrence: 60% of patients with recurrence had received any immunosuppressive drugs and 85.7% of the patients without recurrence.

HLA DR3 is associated with idiopathic MN [36]. In our combined study, HLA DR3 was found in 62% of the patients with MN recurrence, and only in 21% of the patients without recurrence (p = 0.08) [26]. This trend should be evaluated in larger series. No association was found with HLA B8 or HLA B18 and MN recurrence. TAP 1B allele might be a characterised predisposing factor [37] but no data are available on the association with MN recurrence after transplantation.

An association between hepatitis viruses, hepatitis B virus (HBV) and hepatitis C virus (HCV), and MN have been described in native kidneys [38, 39].

In our experience, HBs antigen was present in 20% of the patients with recurrence and 7% of the patients without recurrence but the number of patients was too small in this study to draw any conclusion on a possible association between HBV and recurrent MN.

It has been suggested that MN could be associated with HCV in kidney allografts [40], mainly with *de novo* MN. Morales [40] has described an increased prevalence of *de novo* MN: 15 MGN occurred in 409 HCV positive patients (3.66%) *versus* 0.36% in the HCV negative patients (p < 0.001). There were 2 recurrences, and 3 undetermined GN in the native kidneys. However others series do not confirm this association [39, 41]. In our experience, in kidney transplantation we report an incidence of 1.23% of *de novo* MN in 291 HCV positive patients *versus* 2.43% in HCV negative patients from a cohort of 1,098 patients.

Biologically, MN associated with HCV looks like idiopathic MN, with normal C levels, absence of rheumatoid factor or cryoglobulinemia. Liver function is usually normal at least more often than for patients with MPGN. Most of the patients had an active HCV infection with HCV RNA in their serum.

Pathologically, MN associated with HCV infection was not different from that occurring in HCV negative patients. The clinical outcome of MN associated with HCV infection was similar to that of MN in negative HCV patients [39, 40].

Recipient characteristics after transplantation

Recipient and donor ages were not different in patients with and without MN recurrence.

It has been suggested that MN is more likely to recur in living donor grafts than in cadaveric donor grafts [12, 27, 30, 42]. In the 29 isolated reported cases [26], 13 occurred in recipients from living donors [2, 3, 5, 8, 10-14, 18, 19]. In O'Meara serie [21], on the 23 grafts with recurrence, 16 were from living related and 8 from cadaveric donors, either a prevalence of recurrent glomerulonephritis of 11.9% in the living-related group and 1.3% in the cadaveric donors group (p < 0.001). A similar but non significant increase was reported by Morzycka [18].

Those data prompted some authors to restrict the use of living donors for MN. It is difficult to distinguish between the respective role of the genetic background and of HLA matching in the recurrence.

However, in our combined series [26], the recurrence rate of MN was not significantly different between CD grafts (7/26) and LD grafts (1/4). Those findings were confirmed by the data from the Renal Allograft Disease Registry (RADR) [28]. Mathew *et al.* [43] reported no effect of HLA matching on the recurrence rate.

In the published case reports [2-4, 8, 12-14, 18, 19], the recurrent MN occurred as well in HLA identical patients as in haplo-identical patients. In our own experience in patients receiving a kidney from cadaver donor, we did not find any difference in the degree of HLA A, B and DR matching in patients with and without recurrence [23].

The high rate of recurrence in LD grafts might reflect the lack of competing graft loss from rejection in well matched recipients exposed to relatively long follow-up or the role of HLA matching in favoring recurrence.

Pretransplant native nephrectomy did not prevent or delay the onset of recurrent glomerulonephritis in the renal allograft. The risk of subsequent graft failure from recurrent MN was even higher in the group of patients with pretransplant native nephrectomy [25].

Immunosuppressive therapy after transplantation and membranous nephropathy recurrence

In most of the published cases, cyclosporine A was unable to prevent MN recurrence and *de novo* MN in kidney transplant recipients [12, 20, 25]. In our combined series [23, 26], 4 patients out of the 16 with cyclosporine A had a MN recurrence *versus* 4 out of the 14 patients under conventional therapy with steroids and azathioprine and thus cyclosporine A was unable to prevent or decrease the MN recurrence.

Cyclosporine A is associated with a decreased graft loss due to acute rejection and increased one year-graft survival. This could potentially increase the number of patients with a functioning kidney and their risk of development of recurrent disease [44].

The rate of recurrence was not significantly different in patients receiving antilymphocyte globulins or OKT3 as an induction therapy [23].

No data are available on the possible preventive effect of new immunosuppressive drugs, such as tacrolimus or mycophenolate or rapamycine in the recurrence of glomerular disease, especially MN recurrence.

Outcome of recurrent membranous nephropathy

In the RADR, the actuarial graft survival of patients with recurrent disease is lower than in patients without recurrence [28]. The proportion of graft failure attributable to recurrence *versus* other causes increased from 4.5% at 1 year to over 15% on long term follow-up. The relative risk for graft failure due to recurrent and *de novo* diseases was 1.9 (1.57-2.40) ($p < 0.0001$) in a cohort of 4,913 kidney transplant recipients. The relative risk of graft failure in patients with MN was not significant ($p = 0.13$) while the RR for hemolytic and uremic disease was the highest (RR = 5.36 (2.2-12.9); $p < 0.0002$), followed by MPGN (RR = 2.37 (1.3-4.2; $p < 0.003$), and FSGS (RR = 2.25 (1.6-3.1); $p < 0.0001$) [28].

During the follow-up of at least one year, 55% of the patients with recurrent or *de novo* diseases had a graft failure *versus* 25% of the patients without recurrence or *de novo* diseases (p < 0.0001), although the graft survival rates were not significantly different for the first 2 years.

In the combined study of Lyon and Bruxelles [26], 6 out of the 8 patients with recurrence lost their graft in a mean time of 73 months after transplantation. The outcome of kidney grafts in patients with recurrence was poorer than in patients without recurrence, however not significantly: the actuarial graft loss rate at 5 and 10 years was 38% and 52% respectively in patients with recurrence *versus* 11% and 21% in patients without recurrence. These data have also been found in other studies [8].

The outcome of previously reported cases was poor with a graft loss of 72% at 5 years but these data are biased by the selection of cases with a poor prognosis [26].

Graft loss would occur more rapidly in recurrent MN than in *de novo* MN.

In 33 HLA identical living related donor grafts, with GN as the original disease, the cumulative incidence of recurrence was of 45% at 12 years after transplantation and recurrent GN was the main cause of graft failure [45]. The impact of recurrent disease on graft survival will become more prominent with longer follow-up.

However, MN recurrence was often associated with chronic rejection which seemed to be a major contributing factor in graft loss [7, 11, 23, 46].

Sometimes, the evolution may be favourable, as in native kidneys, with a complete regression of the proteinuria and a disappearance of the histological lesions on a sequential biopsy as we have seen in a patient with a renal graft biopsy performed 3 years after the first one.

Recurrent membranous nephropathy in second kidney grafts

Recurrence of MN in subsequent transplants is possible [16, 17, 47]. The prognosis of this recurrence is unpredictable.

A recurrent crescentic MN in 2 successive renal transplants, associated with choroidal effusions and retinal detachment has been reported in a 50-year old man. Both recurrences led rapidly to renal failure [48]. We previously reported 2 patients who lost their first grafts due to recurrence and chronic rejection in the first one, 141 months after transplantation and from MN recurrence in the second one, 45 months after transplantation. These two patients received a CD graft, 28 and 25 months respectively after the failure of the first graft. The first patient is still alive with a functioning graft while the other developed proteinuria 7 months after the second Tx and graft biopsy showed a recurrent grade 1MN.

Very few data are available on the rate of repeated MN recurrence in the successive grafts. The risk of repeated recurrence is higher in successive grafts than in first grafts and is estimated to 50% for MN, 60% for MPGN and 80% to 100% for FSGS [47]. The risk is the highest in patients who had an early recurrence in the first graft but no risk factors have been identified. As in the first grafts, cyclosporine A is unable to prevent recurrence in second tranplants [16, 17, 48] since the 4 reported cases were under cyclosporine A. Treatment of recurrence with increased immunosuppression seems unhelpful [16].

Recurrence of *de novo* membranous nephropathy after transplantation

A definitive diagnosis of the native kidney disease is required before *de novo* MN can be diagnosed. The incidence of *de novo* MN in the allograft is higher than that of recurrent MN, with more than 7,100 cases reported since the first case described in 1973 by Murphy [30]. Its precise incidence is difficult to know and is estimated at 1-2% of all the transplants [35]. A high incidence of *de novo* MN has been reported in children, around 9.3% of all transplants [49]; however in the 29 children, 7 were HBs antigen positive and 9 cases were detected in routine biopsy specimens. A recurrent *de novo* MN has been described in an adult patient [50]. Out of 7 patients with *de novo* MN on the first graft who were retransplanted, 4 had a recurrent *de novo* MN and those *de novo* MN were seen only in patients with previous *de novo* MN [32]. HLA matching was not better in renal transplant patients who recurred their *de novo* MN on the second graft. HLA DR3 was present in 1 of the 4 patients with recurrent *de novo* MN [32]. *De novo* MN has been described in a conjoint twins [51]. A genetic control of the immune response is probably involved in the ability to develop a *de novo* MN in the allograft. This underlines the importance of host factors in the development of this nephropathy.

De novo MN is frequently accompanied, and often predated by the histological changes of chronic rejection [35]. Nephrotic syndrome is associated with a poor evolution and associated chronic rejection is the major factor determining the prognosis. Cyclosporine A did not change the incidence of *de novo* MN: 9.3% under conventional therapy and 8.6% with cyclosporine A [32, 35]. Little information is available on response to treatment and increasing the dose of oral steroids was unsuccessful in modifying the course of the disease in children [49] while the use of high-dose alternate-day oral steroids was successful in inducing remission of the nephrotic syndrome in one of 3 adults [49]. The pathogenesis of *de novo* MN is unclear: involvement of either an exogeneous antigen or of an alloantigen brought by the graft or of a renal antigen against which an autoantibody develops, or even of an auto-antibody acting as a planted antigen. The presence of antibodies directed against an allogenic tubular epithelial antigen could be involved, sparing the native kidneys. Autologous IgG could play the role of antigen, acting as a planted antigen leading to the formation of immune complexes. Some cases have been reported of an association between *de novo* MN and urologic complications but until now, there is no clear evidence of a causal link between the two events [15].

Urinary excretion C5b-9 reflects disease activity in passive Heymann nephritis [52], but there is no data on the pronostic factor of this marker in *de novo* or recurrent MN in the allograft.

Treatment of recurrent membranous nephropathy

Reported attemps to treat recurrent MN are disappointing. In 3 patients, proteinuria was not affected by the replacement of azathioprine by cyclophosphamide [12, 26].

Methylprednisolone (MP) pulses are unsuccessful [19] although anecdotal remission of nephrotic syndrome in recurrent MN has been achieved with pulsed MP and high dose alternate – day steroids [53]. Treatment by cyclosporine A was unable to prevent and to cure MN [20, 22, 23]. In most of the cases increasing immunosuppressive drugs did not influence the evolution of nephropathy [24].

There is no data available on the efficacy of the replacement of azathioprine by mycophenolate mofetil, or of cyclosporine A by tacrolimus or of the use of rapamycine to treat recurrent MN.

Low-density lipoprotein apheresis combined with simvastatin has been shown partially efficent to decrease proteinuria due to MN in the allograft [54].

Protein A immunoadsorption is efficient in nephrotic syndrome of various etiologies but has a transient effect [55].

Symptomatic treatment of nephrotic syndrome, especially ACE inhibitors, is recommended in recurrent MN, as in native kidneys.

In conclusion, recurrent MN occurs in 25% of the patients who received a kidney for MN. The pathogenesis is unclear. No predictive risk factor has been identified and immunosuppressive drugs given after transplantation, especially cyclosporine A, are unable to prevent MN recurrence. There is no recognised specific treatment.

References

1. Crosson JT, Wathen RL, Raij L, Andersen RC, Anderson WR. Recurrence of idiopathic membranous nephropathy in a renal allograft. *Arch Intern Med* 1975; 135: 1101-6.
2. Petersen VP, Olsen TS, Kissmeyer-Nielsen F, Bohman S-O, Hansen HE, Hansen ES, Skov PE, Solling K. Late failure of human renal transplants. An analysis of transplant disease and graft failure among 125 recipients surviving for one to eight years. *Medicine* 1975; 54: 45-69.
3. Rubin RJ, Pinn VW, Barnes BA, Harrington JT. Recurrent idiopathic membranous glomerulonephritis. *Transplantation* 1977; 24: 4-9.
4. Hills GS, Robertson J, Grossman R, Perloff L, Barker CF. An unusual variant of membranous nephropathy with abundant crescent formation and recurrence in the transplanted kidney. *Clin Nephrol* 1978; 10: 114-20.
5. Lieberthal W, Bernard DB, Donohoe JE, Stilmant MM, Couser WG. Rapid recurrence of membranous nephropathy in a related renal allograft. *Clin Nephrol* 1979; 12: 222-8.
6. Briner J, Binswanger U, Largiader F. Recurrent and *de novo* membranous glomerulonephritis in renal cadaver allotransplants. *Clin Nephrol* 1980; 13: 189-96.
7. Dische FE, Herbertson BM, Melcher DH, Morley AR. Membranous glomerulonephritis in transplant kidneys: recurrent or *de novo* disease in four patients. *Clin Nephrol* 1981; 15: 154-63.
8. Iskandar SS, Jennette JC. Recurrence of membranous glomerulopathy in an allograft. Case report and review of the literature. *Nephron* 1981; 29: 270-3.
9. Verani R, Dan M. Membranous glomerulonephritis in renal transplant: a case report and review of the literature. *Am J Nephrol* 1982; 2: 316-20.
10. First MR, Mendoza N, Maryniak RK, Weiss MA. Membranous glomerulopathy following kidney transplantation. Association with renal vein thrombosis in two of nine cases. *Transplantation* 1984; 38: 603-7.
11. Honkanen E, Törnroth T, Pettersson E, Kuhlbäck B. Glomurelonephritis in renal allografts: results of 18 years of transplantation. *Clin Nephrol* 1984; 21: 210-9.
12. Obermiller LE, Hoy WE, Eversole M, Sterling WA. Recurrent membranous glomurelonephritis in two renal transplants. *Transplantation* 1985; 40: 100-2.
13. Freedman BI, Graves JW, Burkart JM, Callahan MF, Tell GS, Heis ER, Adams PL. The impact of different immunosuppressant regimens on recurrent glomerulonephritis. *Transplant Proc* 1989; 21: 2121-2.

14. Agarwal SK, Dash SC, Mehta SN, Bhuyan UN. Recurrence of idiopathic membranous nephropathy in HLA-identical allograft. *Nephron* 1992; 60: 366.
15. Robles NR, Gomez-Campdera F, Anaya F, Niembro E, Valderrabano F. Membranous glomerulonephritis after kidney transplantation and urologic complications. *Am J Nephrol* 1992; 12: 279-80.
16. Innes A, Woodrow G, Boyd SM, Beckingham IJ, Morgan AG. Recurrent membranous nephropathy in successive renal transplants. *Nephrol Dial Transplant* 1994; 9: 323-5.
17. Josephson MA, Spargo B, Hollandsworth D, Thistlethwaite JR. The recurrence of recurrent membranous glomerulopathy in a renal transplant recipient: case report and literature review. *Am J Kidney Dis* 1994; 24: 873-8.
18. Morzycka M, Croker BP Jr, Seigler HF, Tischer CC. Evaluation of recurrent glomerulonephritis in kidney allografts. *Am J Med* 1982; 72: 588-98.
19. Berger BE, Vincenti F, Biava C, Amend WJ Jr, Feduska N, Salvatierra O Jr. De novo and recurrent membranous glomerulopathy following kidney transplantation. *Transplantation* 1983; 35: 315-9.
20. Montagnino G, Colturi C, Banfi G, Aroldi A, Tarantino A, Ponticelli C. Membranous nephropathy in cyclosporine-treated renal transplant recipients. *Transplantation* 1989; 47: 725-7.
21. O'Meara Y, Green A, Carmody M, Donohoe J, Campbell E, Browne O, Walshe J. Recurrent glomerulonephritis in renal transplants: fourteen years' experience. *Nephrol Dial Transplant* 1989; 4: 730-4.
22. Schwarz A, Krause PH, Offermann G, Keller F. Recurrent and de novo renal disease after kidney transplantation with or without cyclosporine A. *Am J Kidney Dis* 1991; 17: 524-31.
23. Couchoud C, Pouteil-Noble C, Colon S, Touraine JL. Recurrence of membranous nephropathy after renal transplantation. *Transplantation* 1995; 59: 1275-9.
24. Marcen R, Mampaso F, Teruel JL, Rivera ME, Orofino L, Navarro-Antolin J, Ortuno J. Membranous nephropathy; recurrence after kidney transplantation. *Nephrol Dial Transplant* 1996; 11: 1129-33.
25. Odorico JS, Knechtle SJ, Rayhill SC, Pirsch JD, D'Alessandro AM, Belzer FO, Sollinger HW. The influence of native nephrectomy on the incidence of recurrent disease following renal transplantation for primary glomerulonephritis. *Transplantation* 1996; 61: 228-34.
26. Cosyns JP, Couchoud C, Pouteil-Noble C, Squifflet JP, Pirson Y. Recurrence of membranous nephropathy after renal transplantation: probability, outcome and risk factors. *Clin Nephrol* 1998; 50: 144-53.
27. Mathew TH. Recurrence of disease following renal transplantation. *Am J Kidney Dis* 1988; 12: 85-96.
28. Hariharan S, Adams MB, Brennan DC, et al. Recurrent and de novo glomerular disease after renal transplantation. *Transplantation* 1999; 68: 635-41.
29. Baqi N, Tejani A. Recurrence of the original disease in pediatric renal transplantation. *J Nephrol* 1997; 10: 85-92.
30. Davison AM, Johnston PA. Allograft membranous nephropathy. *Nephrol Dial Transplant* 1992; (Suppl. 1): 114-8
31. Ehrenreich T, Porush JG, Churg J, Garfinkel L, Glabman S, Goldstein MII, Grishmann E, Yunis SL. Treatment of idiopathic membranous nephropathy. *N Engl J Med* 1976; 295: 741-6.
32. Heidet L, Gagnadoux MF, Beziau A, Niaudet P, Broyer M, Habib R. Recurrence of de novo membranous glomerulonephritis on renal grafts. *Clin Nephrol* 1994; 41: 314-8.
33. Broyer M, Selwood N, Brunner F. Recurrence of primary renal disease on kidney graft: a European pediatric experience. *J Am Soc Nephrol* 1992; 2: 255-7.
34. Müller T, Sikora P, Offner G, Hoyer PF, Brodehl J. Recurrence of renal disease after kidney transplantation in children: 24 years of experience in a single center. *Clin Nephrol* 1998; 49: 82-90.
35. Schwarz A, Krause PH, Offerman G, Keller F. Impact of de novo memebranous glomerulonephritis on the clinical course after kidney transplantation. *Transplantation* 1994; 58: 650-4.
36. Klouda PT, Manos J, Acheson EJ, Dyer PA, Goldby FS, Harris R, Lawier W, Mallick NP, Williams G. Strong association between idiopathic membranous nephropathy and HLA-DRW3. *Lancet* 1979; 2: 770-1.
37. Chevrier D, Giral M, Braud V, Soulillou JP, Bignon JD. Membranous nephropathy and a TAP1 gene polymorphism. *N Engl J Med* 1994; 331: 133-4.
38. Johnson RJ, Couser WG. Hepatitis B infection and renal disease: clinical, immunopathogenetic and therapeutic considerations. *Kidney Int* 1990; 37: 663-76.
39. Pouteil-Noble C, Maiza H, Dijoud F, Mac Grégor B. Glomerular disease associated with hepatitis C virus infection in native kidneys. *Nephrol Dial Transplant* 2000; 15 (Suppl. 8): 28-33.
40. Morales JM, Pascual-Capdevila J, Campistol JM, et al. Membranous glomerulonephritis associated with hepatitis C virus infection in renal transplant patients. *Transplantation* 1997; 63: 1634-9.
41. Hammoud H, Haem J, Laurent B, et al. Glomerular disease during HCV infection in renal transplantation. *Nephrol Dial Transplant* 1996; 11 (Suppl. 4): 54-5.

42. Dantal J, Giral M, Hourmant M, Soulillou JP. Glomerulonephritis recuurences after kidney transplantation. *Curr Opin Nephrol Hypertens* 1995; 4: 146-54.
43. Mathew TH, Mathews DC, Hobbs JB, Kincaid-Smith P. Glomerular lesions after renal transplantation. *Am J Med* 1975; 59: 177-90.
44. Ramos EL, Tisher CC. Recurrent diseases in the kidney transplant. *Am J Kidney Dis* 1994; 1: 142-54.
45. Andresdottir MB, Hoitsma AJ, Assman KJM, Koene RAP, Wetzels JFM. The impact of recurrent glomerulonephritis on graft survival in recipients of human histocompatibility leucocyte antigen-identical living related donor grafts. *Transplantation* 1999; 68: 623-7.
46. Truong L, Gelfand J, D'Agati V, Tomaszewski J, Appel G, Hardy M, Pirani CL. De novo membranous glomerulonephropathy in renal allografts: a report of ten cases and review of the literature. *Am J Kidney Dis* 1989; 14: 131-44.
47. De Meyer M, Pouteil-Noble C, Peeters J, Cosyns JP, McGregor B, Vanrenterghem Y, Touraine JL, Squifflet JP, Pirson Y. The fate of second kidney transplant after recurrence of glomerulonephritis in the first transplant. In: *Retransplantation, transplantation and clinical immunology*, 29th ed. Kluwer Academic Publishers: 29-38.
48. Lazowski P, Sablay LB, Glicklich D. Recurrent crescentic membranous nephropathy in 2 successive renal transplants: association with choroidal effusions and retinal detachment. *Am J Nephrol* 1998; 18: 146-50.
49. Antignac C, Hinglais N, Gubler MC, Gagnadoux MF, Broyer M, Habib R. De novo membranous glomerulonephritis in renal allografts in children. *Clin Nephrol* 1988; 30: 1-7.
50. Cosyns JP, Pirson Y, Van Ypersele de Strihou C, Alexandre GPJ. Recurrence of de novo graft membranous glomerulonephritis. *Nephron* 1981; 29: 142-5.
51. Bansal VK, Kozeny GA, Fresco R, Vertuno LL, Hano JE. De novo membranous nephropathy following renal transplantation between conjoint twins. *Transplantation* 1986; 41: 404-6.
52. Pruchno CJ, Burns MW, Schulze M, Johnson R, Baker PJ, Couser W. Urinary excretion of C5b-C9 reflects disease activity in passive Heymann nephritis. *Kidney Int* 1989; 36: 65-71.
53. Johnston PA, Goode NP, Aparicio SR, Davison AM. Membranous allograft nephropathy. Remission of nephrotic syndrome with pulsed methylprednisolone and high-dose alternate-day steroids. *Transplantation* 1993; 55: 214-6.
54. Ideura T, Hora K, Kaneko Y, Yamazaki T, Tokunaga S, Shigematsu H, Kiyosawa K. Effect of low-density liporotein-apheresis on nephrotic syndrome due to membranous nephropathy in renal allograft: a case report. *Transplant Proc* 2000; 32: 223-6.
55. Esnault V, Besnier D, Testa A, Coville P, Simon P, Subra JF, Audrain MAP. Effect of protein A immunoadsorption in nephrotic syndrome of various etiologies. *J Am Soc Nephrol* 1999; 10: 2014-7.
56. Lustig S, Yussim A, Shmueli D, *et al*. Recurrent and de novo glomerulopathies after renal transplantation. Possible beneficial effect of cyclosporin in FSGS and MPGN (Abstract). XIIIth Int Congress Nephrol Jerusalem, 1993.

Recurrent IgA nephropathy after kidney transplantation

Jürgen Floege
Division of Nephrology, University of Aachen, Germany

IgA nephropathy (IgAN) is the most common type of glomerulonephritis in the Western world [1]. Affected patients usually represent ideal candidates for a renal graft and therefore account for a significant share of transplant patients. Unfortunately, it was quickly realized that up to 60% of the patients will experience a histological recurrence of the disease [2]. Until recently, it has been assumed that the histological recurrence of IgAN after transplantation is a relatively benign condition and hardly ever affects the graft function. This view has been challenged by several recent studies [2-8], which will be summarized below.

The major problem in studying the origin of graft failure in patients with underlying IgAN is that it may be very difficult to separate the clinical relevance of recurrent IgAN from other mechanisms of chronic graft failure. By definition, the diagnosis of recurrent IgAN requires an accurate identification and characterization of glomerulonephritis in the native kidneys and subsequent identification of the same disease affecting the transplant kidney. Of note, these basic requirements are often not fulfilled in reports in the literature. In the case of recurrent IgAN detailed clinical data and biopsy findings (in particular when examined by immunohistology and electron microscopy as well) can usually allow with some likelihood to differentiate between the relative contribution of dysfunction due to recurrent disease and other reasons, in particular the so-called "chronic rejection". Clinically manifest recurrent IgAN is often associated with persistent microhematuria and proteinuria exceeding 0.5 g/day. Histologically this should be associated with the demonstration of mesangioproliferative glomerulonephritis, *i.e.* not just recurrent mesangial IgA deposits, in the graft.

In recent years, seven retrospective, single-center studies have assessed the clinical relevance of recurrent IgAN [2-8] *(Table I)*. Importantly, mean follow-up in all of these studies was longer than 5 years. This may explain why earlier, more short-term studies failed to detect a clinical impact of recurrent disease, since recurrence related graft deterioration is rare before 3 years after transplantation. In the seven recent studies, the clear message evolved that recurrent IgAN becomes clinically relevant and significantly contributes to graft failure once a 5 year follow-up has passed. At this time between 11% and 23% of all patients exhibited some recurrence-related graft dysfunction and between 2% and 16% had lost their graft due to recurrence *(Table I)*. In our own study [5], it also became apparent that the impact of recurrent IgAN may be diluted by

Table I. Summary of recent studies on the clinical relevance of recurrent IgAN after transplantation (modified from [14])

Authors	Patients n =	Follow-up in the whole study population (mean and range; months)	Graft dysfunction/ loss due to recurrence	Follow-up in patients with graft dysfunction/loss due to recurrence of IgAN (mean and range; months)
Odum et al. 1994 [2]	46	n.a. (3-183)	11%/2%	62 (32-75)
Kessler et al. 1996[a] [3]	28[a]	73 (4-120)[a]	21%/14%	84 (43-119)
Frohnert et al. 1997 [4]	51	n.a. (< 3-> 156)	19%16%	n.a. (12- > 144)
Ohmacht et al. 1997 [5]	61[b]	54 (7-127)	23%/16%	67 (32-102)
Bumgardner et al. 1998 [6]	54	61 (n.a.)	16%/10%	75 (n.a.)
Freese et al. 1999 [7]	104[c]	67[d] (11-159)	13%/6%	n.a.
Kim et al. 2001 [8]	89	60 (2-164)	n.a./2%	n.a.

[a] Only patients who received a transplant biopsy because of graft dysfunction or urinary abnormalities are included in the data shown. Five patients suffered from underlying Henoch-Schönlein purpura.
[b] Four patients suffered from underlying Henoch-Schönlein purpura.
[c] 50% of the patients had living donors.
[d] Median and range.
n.a.: Not available.

the more rapid manifestation of chronic allograft rejection and/or other reasons for graft failure. Another important finding was that, out of five patients who were re-transplanted after graft failure due to recurrent IgAN, three again developed end stage renal disease at 21-51 months due to repeated recurrence of the primary disease. Thus, patients who have already lost a graft due to recurrent IgAN may be at particularly high risk for repeated graft loss due to recurrence upon re-transplantation.

In contrast to recurrent IgAN, much less is known on the course of Henoch-Schönlein purpura (HSP), considered by many to represent the systemic variant of IgAN, after renal transplantation. The data available up to date suggest that recurrence of clinically relevant IgAN in patients with underlying HSP is similar to that observed in patients with underlying IgAN [5, 9]. The only large study published also suggests that delaying transplantation until 1 year after the disappearance of purpura has no effect on the recurrence rate [9].

With respect to predictors of clinically relevant recurrent IgAN, it appears to represent largely a function of time post-transplantation and cannot be predicted by other variables. In this respect, the recurrent disease exhibits considerable clinical similarities with the original course of progressive IgAN. All recent studies [2-8] consistently demonstrated that neither clinical and laboratory findings prior to transplantation, the HLA-typing or matching, the ACE I/D-gene polymorphism, the type of immunosuppression nor the course after renal transplantation was able to predict graft failure due to recurrent IgAN. Recent data from the Mayo Clinic [4] and from Korea [8] also do not support earlier Swedish data [7] that living-related donor transplantation should be discouraged in patients with IgAN, as these grafts exhibited no higher rates of recurrence or failure than cadaveric transplants.

Should transplantation potentially be discouraged in patients with underlying IgAN? Long term stable courses of up to 183 months even in the face of histologically proven IgAN recurrence have been documented after transplantation [2-8]. Compared to many other patients suffering from systemic disorders who enter dialysis, those with IgAN generally have little co-morbidity and as such present ideal candidates for transplantation. Graft and patient survival in the first years after transplantation is reported to be superior to that of other transplant patients, possibly related to the increased occurrence of alloreactive IgA anti-HLA antibodies in such patients and their overreactivity of the IgA system. These IgA anti-HLA antibodies may be be less pathogenic than IgG anti-HLA antibodies [10]. Finally, at least one study documented that patient and graft survival up to ten years after grafting in case of an underlying IgAN is not different from that observed in patients with other types of glomerulonephritis or non-glomerulonephritic disorders leading to end stage renal disease [8]. Given all these observations, primary IgAN definitely should not prevent transplantation. However, it appears important that both physicians as well as patients with underlying IgAN (particularly those who have already lost a graft due to recurrence) are aware of the fact that recurrent disease may cause graft loss after about 5 years onward.

Currently, there is no established treatment to prevent recurrence of IgAN after transplantation. In this respect, the recent introduction of mycophenolate mofetil (MMF) into clinical transplantation offers some hope. MMF, unlike currently available immunosuppressive agents, has considerable activity on B-lymphocytes in addition to T-lymphocytes and may thereby reduce the exaggerated IgA production in IgAN patients. Also, recent data suggest that MMF has direct anti-proliferative on mesangial cells *in vivo* [11]. Finally, Nowack *et al.* [12] describe a case of a patient with recurrent, progressive IgAN following transplantation, in whom the institution of MMF therapy led to a stabilization of the course. Unfortunately, all other data available up to date on MMF in patients with underlying IgAN suffer from short-term follow-up and it will therefore take several years to establish the role of this potential new approach for the prevention of recurrent IgAN. Until then, we are left with more conventional approaches to prevent progression of renal failure, in particular the usage of ACE-inhibitors in such patients [13].

References

1. Floege J, Feehally J. IgA nephropathy: recent developments. *J Am Soc Nephrol* 2000; 11: 2395-403.
2. Odum J, Peh CA, Clarkson AR, Bannister KM, Seymour AE, Gillis D, Thomas AC, Mathew TH, Woodroffe AJ. Recurrent mesangial IgA nephritis following renal transplantation. *Nephrol Dial Transplant* 1994; 9: 309-12.
3. Kessler M, Hiesse C, Hestin D, Mayeux D, Boubenider K, Charpentier B. Recurrence of immunoglobulin A nephropathy after renal transplantation in the cyclosporine era. *Am J Kidney Dis* 1996; 28: 99-104.
4. Frohnert PP, Donadio JV Jr, Velosa JA, Holley KE, Sterioff S. The fate of renal transplants in patients with IgA nephropathy. *Clin Transplant* 1997; 11: 127-33.
5. Ohmacht C, Kliem V, Burg M, Nashan B, Schlitt HJ, Brunkhorst R, Koch KM, Floege J. Recurrent immunoglobulin A nephropathy after renal transplantation: a significant contributor to graft loss. *Transplantation* 1997; 64: 1493-6.
6. Bumgardner GL, Amend WC, Ascher NL, Vincenti FG. Single-center long-term results of renal transplantation for IgA nephropathy. *Transplantation* 1998; 65: 1053-60.

AS is caused by an inherited defect in type-IV collagen chains. In approximately 85% of AS pedigrees, the disease is X-linked and mutations identified so far are in the COL4A5 gene. In the majority of non-X-linked families, transmission appears to be autosomal recessive with mutations detected in either the COL4A3 or the COL4A4 gene. In most males with COL4A5 mutations, α3 (IV) and α4 (IV) chains, as well as α5 (IV) chains are not expressed in the GBM. These three chains are similarly absent from the GBM in most patients with COL4A3 or COL4A4 mutation. It is thought that an abnormality in one of the three chains limits the formation of the triple helice, thereby preventing incorporation of the two others into GBM [4]. AS patients who develop anti-GBM disease in the allograft presumably fail to develop immunologic tolerance for these chains [4]. Not surprisingly, these allo-antibodies are directed to α3 (IV), α4 (IV) and α5 (IV) chains [5-9].

Recent experimental evidence indicates that both auto – and allo – anti-GBM antibodies bind rapidly to α3 (IV)NC1 domain and remain tightly bound, with slow dissociation rates. This property likely contributes to both the fulminant nature of the disease and its resistance to therapy [10].

Recurrence of anti-GBM disease in the kidney graft

Anti-GBM disease has an estimated incidence of one case per 2 million, per year, in the European Caucasoid population [11]. Glomerulonephritis may be associated or not with lung hemorrhage (Goodpasture syndrome). In general, glomerulonephritis progresses rapidly, resulting in ESRF in about 70% of cases. Though treatment with plasma exchange and immunosuppression is generally successful in patients presenting with a serum creatinine below 5 mg/dl, recovery of renal function is very unlikely in patients with dialysis-dependent renal failure at presentation [11]. The affected patients are usually young, so that most of them are eligible for renal transplantation (TP). According to the EDTA-ERA Registry, 0.5% of renal TP recorded between 1982 and 1990 have been performed in patients with anti-GBM nephritis [12].

Recurrence of anti-GBM disease in the kidney graft is now a rare event. Histological recurrence of anti-GBM nephritis in the graft has been documented in up to 55% of patients as long as anti-GBM antibodies monitoring was not available [13]. Subsequently, it became the rule to delay TP until disappearance of circulating anti-GBM antibodies – determined by a sensitive assay (Elisa or RIA) – for at least 6 to 12 months; clinical recurrence then became very rare (even claimed to be reduced to zero) [14].

In order to better document the risk of recurrence, we have reviewed the outcome of 21 TP performed between January 1977 and December 2000 in the Cliniques Universitaires St. Luc, Brussels, in 19 patients (11 men, 8 women; mean age at the time of TP: 39 years, range 18-62) with anti-GBM disease. Anti-GBM nephritis was defined by crescentic glomerulonephritis (n = 18) or end-stage kidney (n = 1) with linear glomerular IgG and/or circulating anti-GBM antibodies. Duration of dialysis ranged from 4 to 179 (mean 34) months. At the time of TP, anti-GBM antibodies had vanished in all previously positive patients for a mean of 26 (3-131) months. Currently, 2 to 181 (mean 95) months after the first TP, 18 patients are alive, 14 of whom with a functioning graft. Seventeen out of 19 transplanted patients (88%) had no clinical sign of recurrence.

A graft biopsy was performed in 7 of them for graft dysfunction. There was no Ig deposit in 6 of them. In the last one, a linear IgG deposit along the GBM was disclosed 2 months after TP, without associated glomerular injury and in the absence of circulating anti-GBM antibodies; currently, 5 years later, this graft has an adequate function. Recurrence of anti-GBM disease occurred in the remaining two patients. The first, transplanted after 28 months of dialysis, developed proteinuria and hematuria 14 months after TP. Recurrence of anti-GBM disease was demonstrated by linear IgA (without IgG) deposits on 3 successive biopsies, with crescentic glomerulonephritis. Despite substitution of cyclophosphamide for azathioprine, graft function deteriorated, leading to resumption of dialysis 55 months after TP. Interestingly, circulating IgG and IgA anti-GBM antibodies were never detected despite IgG and IgA deposits in the native kidneys and IgA deposits in the graft. A second TP, performed 5 months later, has currently an adequate function, 59 months later. In the last patient, reported elsewhere (15) anti-GBM nephritis recurred – with reappearance of anti-GBM antibodies – after the spontaneous withdrawal of immunosuppressive treatment more than 5 years after TP. Treatment with cyclophosphamide and methylprednisolone was unsuccessful, and dialysis was resumed.

Several lessons may be learned from this experience. First, the overall good prognosis of TP in patients with anti-GBM nephritis is confirmed, with no clinical recurrence in 94% of patients complying with their post-TP immunosuppressive regimen. Second, recurrence of linear Ig staining on the GBM is not necessarily accompanied by histological or clinical glomerulonephritis and is compatible with a good prognosis. Third, clinical recurrence can nevertheless occur, despite a pre-TP waiting time of more than 2 years without detectable anti-GBM antibodies in the serum. Fourth, IgA anti-GBM nephritis might represent a rare subset of the disease more prone to recurrence. Fifth, withdrawal of immunosuppressive treatment can trigger recurrence, even after a prolonged period of quiescence. This challenges the concept of anti-GBM nephritis as a single-shot illness and suggests that maintenance immunosuppressive therapy may help suppress auto-antibody production [15].

Taken together, these observations should not preclude renal TP in any patient with anti-GBM nephritis, provided anti-GBM antibodies are no longer detected in the circulation, preferably for at least 6 months [1].

De novo anti-GBM disease in patients with Alport's syndrome

AS has an estimated prevalence of 1:5,000 to 1:10,000. The disease is characterized by a progressive glomerulonephritis erratically associated with various extra-renal features, mainly sensorineural deafness and ocular abnormalities (retinal flecks, anterior lenticonus and recurrent corneal erosions) [16]. The risk of progression to ESRF is highest among males with the X-linked form and among patients of both sexes with the autosomal recessive form. AS accounts for 1 to 2% of cases of ESRF in Western countries [16].

The risk to develop anti-GBM nephritis in the kidney graft is lower than previous estimates, ranging from 3 to 10% [4, 17]. From a total of 94 AS patients transplanted in four centers [18-21], crescentic anti-GBM nephritis actually occurred in only two cases, *i.e.* a rate of 2%. Such a low prevalence explains that recurrence does not impact overall results of TP in AS patients: as documented in Brussels [20] and Hamburg [21] as well as in US and European registries [22, 23], graft survival rates in AS patients do not differ from those of patients with other primary nephropathies.

Unfortunately, graft prognosis in the few patients experiencing recurrence is extremely poor since anti-GBM nephritis led to graft loss within a few weeks to months in 75% of patients, despite treatment with cyclophosphamide and plasmapheresis in some of them [17]. The clinical and genetic profile of 26 patients developing this complication has been drawn by Kashtan [22]. Roughly, 88% were hemizygotes with severe X-linked disease and 12% were homozygotes with the autosomal-recessive form; no case has been documented so far in heterozygous females with the X-linked form. All patients were deaf and 96% had reached ESRF before the age of 30. The mutation responsible for AS has been identified in 12 patients: it was located in the COL4A5 gene in 9 males (7 complete or partial deletions; one splice-site mutation; one missense mutation) and in the COL4A3 gene in 3 females [22, 24]. Remarkably, all these mutations but one are predicted to result in a truncated $\alpha 5$ or $\alpha 3(IV)$ chain lacking the NC1 domain, an observation which is in line with the pathogenic hypothesis of a congenital failure to develop immune tolerance to critical epitopes in $\alpha 5/\alpha 3(IV)$ chains *(see above)*.

Truncating mutations in AS genes thus predispose to post-TP anti-GBM nephritis: as regard to the COL4A5 gene, a large deletion was indeed found in 50% of 14 patients with post-TP anti-GBM nephritis screened for a COL4A5 mutation, as compared with a deletion frequency of at most 16% in the general AS population [5]. Still, the majority of patients with a large deletion in the COL4A5 gene did not develop post-TP anti-GBM nephritis [5, 25, 26]. Moreover, in the same kindred with a COL4A5 deletion, some affected individuals suffered this complication whereas others had an uneventful long-term post-TP course [17]. Clearly, factors other than the type of mutation must be involved in the full-blown development of this complication. Interestingly, linear IgG staining along graft GBM in the absence of proliferative glomerulonephritis has been documented in about 15% of AS patients, suggesting the existence of a mild immunization, insufficient to trigger the cascade of events culminating in crescentic glomerulonephritis [19, 20]. In line with this observation, it has even been demonstrated recently that all AS patients develop anti-GBM antibodies after TP, irrespective of whether they manifest nephritis or not. By using direct Elisa and immunoblotting with (IV)NC1 domains, Kalluri *et al.* indeed detected antibodies variably directed against $\alpha 3/\alpha 4/\alpha 5$ (IV) chains in all post-TP serum samples from 21 AS patients, 10 with and 11 without anti-GBM nephritis. The pattern of antibodies reactivity did not differ between the two groups, suggesting that individual variability in cell-mediated rather than in humoral immune response ultimately determines the development of anti-GBM nephritis [9].

In AS patients in whom a first graft was lost from anti-GBM nephritis, the risk of recurrence in a subsequent graft exceeds 50% and is invariable if anti-GBM antibodies persist at the time of retransplantation [4, 18, 27].

In summary, graft destruction from *de novo* anti-GBM nephritis occurs in 2% of AS patients, almost all of whom have a mutation resulting in the absence of the (IV) NC1 domain. However, since the majority of AS patients harbouring such a mutation do not develop this complication, there is no reason to deny any AS patient a first kidney TP.

By contrast, attempting a second transplant after the loss of the first one from anti-GBM nephritis carries a very high risk of recurrence.

Acknowledgements

To Mrs Madeleine Putmans for secretarial assistance.

References

1. Kluth DC, Rees AJ. Anti-glomerular basement membrane disease. *J Am Soc Nephrol* 1999; 10: 2446-53.
2. Noël LH, Bobrie G, Pochet JM, Pirson Y, Goldman M, Moulonguet-Doleris L, Farge D, Déchelette E, Grünfeld JP. Glomérulonéphrites à anticorps anti-membrane basale glomérulaire (MBG) après transplantation rénale. *Néphrologie* 1989; 10: 113-5.
3. Borza DB, Netzer KO, Leinonen A, Todd P, Cervera J, Saus J, Hudson BG. The Goodpasture Autoantigen. Identification of multiple cryptic epitopes on the NC1 domain of the α3 (IV) collagen chain. *J Biol Chem* 2000; 275: 6030-7.
4. Kashtan CE, Michael AF. Alport syndrome. *Kidney Int* 1996; 50: 1445-63.
5. Ding J, Zhou J, Tryggvason K, Kashtan CE. COL4A5 deletions in three patients with Alport syndrome and postransplant antiglomerular basement membrane nephritis. *J Am Soc Nephrol* 1994; 5: 161-8.
6. Kalluri R, Weber M, Netzer KO, Sun MJ, Neilson EG, Hudson BG. COL4A5 gene deletion and production of post-transplant anti-α3 (IV) collagen alloantibodies in Alport syndrome. *Kidney Int* 1994; 45: 721-6.
7. Dehan P, Van Den Heuvel LPWJ, Smeets HJM, Tryggvason K, Foidart JM. Identification of post-transplant anti-α5 (IV) collagen alloantibodies in X-linked Alport syndrome. *Nephrol Dial Transplant* 1996; 11: 1983-8.
8. Brainwood D, Kashtan C, Gubler MC, Turner AN. Targets of alloantibodies in Alport anti-glomerular basement membrane disease after renal transplantation. *Kidney Int* 1998; 53: 763-6.
9. Kalluri R, Torre A, Shield III CF, Zamborsky ED, Werner MC, Suchin E, Wolf G, Helmchen UM, Van den Heuvel LPWJ, Grossman R, Aradhye S, Neilson EG. Identification of α3, α4, and α5 chains of type IV collagen as alloantigens for Alport posttransplant anti-glomerular basement membrane antibodies. *Transplantation* 2000; 69: 679-82.
10. Rutgers A, Meyers KEC, Canziani G, Kalluri R, Lin J, Madaio MP. High affinity of anti-GBM antibodies from Goodpasture and transplanted Alport patients to α3 (IV)NC1 collagen. *Kidney Int* 2000; 58: 115-22.
11. Levy JB, Turner AN, Rees AJ, Pusey CD. Long-term outcome of anti-glomerular basement membrane antibody disease treated with plasma exchange and immunosuppression. *Ann Intern Med* 2001; 134: 1032-42.
12. Netzer KO, Merkel F, Weber M. Goodpasture syndrome and end-stage renal failure – to transplant or not to transplant? *Nephrol Dial Transplant* 1998; 13: 1346-8.
13. Wilson CB, Dixon FJ. Anti-glomerular basement membrane antibody-induced glomerulonephritis. *Kidney Int* 1973; 3: 74-89.
14. Cameron JS. Recurrent renal disease after renal transplantation. *Curr Opin Nephrol Hypert* 1994; 3: 602-7.
15. Fonck C, Loute G, Cosyns JP, Pirson Y. Recurrent fulminant anti-GBM nephritis at a 7-year interval. *Am J Kidney Dis* 1998; 2: 323-7.
16. Pirson Y. Making the diagnosis of Alport's syndrome. *Kidney Int* 1999; 56: 760-75.
17. Kashtan CE, Butkowski RJ, Kleppel MM, Roy First M, Michael AF. Posttransplant anti-glomerular basement membrane nephritis in related males with Alport syndrome. *J Lab Clin Med* 1990; 116: 508-15.
18. Milliner DS, Pierides AM, Holley KE. Renal transplantation in Alport's syndrome. *Mayo Clin Proc* 1982; 57: 35-43.
19. Querin S, Noël LH, Grünfeld JP, *et al.* Linear glomerular IgG fixation in renal allografts: incidence and significance in Alport's syndrome. *Clin Nephrol* 1986; 25: 134-40.

20. Peten E, Pirson Y, Cosyns JP, Squifflet JP, Alexandre GPJ, Noël LH, Grünfeld JP, van Ypersele C. Outcome of thirty patients with Alport's syndrome after renal transplantation. *Transplantation* 1991; 52: 823-6.
21. Göbel J, Olbricht CJ, Offner G, Helmchen U, Repp H, Koch KM, Frei U. Kidney transplantation in Alport's syndrome: long-term outcome and allograft anti-GBM nephritis. *Clin Nephrol* 1992; 38: 299-304.
22. Kashtan CE, McEnery PT, Tejani A, Stablein DM. Renal allograft survival according to primary diagnosis: a report of the North American Pediatric Renal Transplant Cooperative Study. *Pediatr Nephrol* 1995; 9: 679-84.
23. Ridgen SPA, Mehls O, Jones EHP, Valderrabano F. The child-adult interface: a report on Alport's syndrome, 1975-1993. *Nephrol Dial Transplant* 1996; 11 (Suppl. 7): 21-7.
24. Lemminck HH, Schröder CH, Monnens LAH, Smeets HJM. The clinical spectrum of type IV collagen mutations. *Hum Mutat* 1997; 9: 477-99.
25. Pirson Y, Lannoy N, Smaers M, Tryggvason K, Verellen-Dumoulin C. Deletion in the COL4A5 gene and outcome of renal transplantation in Alport syndrome. *Nephrol Dial Transplant* 1992; 7: 785.
26. Antignac C, Knebelmann B, Druout L, Gros F, Deschenes G, Hors-Cayla MC, Zhou J, Tryggvason K, Grünfeld JP, Broyer M, Gubler MC. Deletions in the COL4A5 collagen gene in X-linked Alport syndrome: characterization of the pathological transcripts in non-renal cells and correlation with disease expression. *J Clin Invest* 1994; 93: 1195-207.
27. Goldman M, Depierreux M, De Pauw L, Vereerstraeten P, Kinnaert P, Noël LH, Grünfeld JP, Toussaint C. Failure of two subsequent renal grafts by anti-GBM glomerulonephritis in Alport's syndrome: case report and review of the literature. *Transplant Int* 1990; 3: 82-5.

Recurrence of the Disease in the Renal Graft
Cochat P, ed.
© John Libbey Eurotext, Paris, 2001

De novo renal diseases after renal transplantation

Sundaram Hariharan
Medical College of Wisconsin, Division of Nephrology, Wilwaukee, USA

Immunosuppressive agents such as cyclosporine, tacrolimus, mycophenolate mofetil and rapamycin have reduced acute rejection rates after renal transplantation, without any impact on recurrent and *de novo* diseases [1]. Development of recurrent or *de novo* disease has been associated with significant graft dysfunction and graft failure on long-term follow-up [2].

Native kidney disease is poorly defined in many patients with end stage renal disease. This poses a problem in identifying and differentiating recurrent and *de novo* disease. By definition recurrent disease is the original kidney disease occurring in the transplanted kidney. *De novo* disease is when new disease develops in the transplanted kidney. *De novo* disease can be of 2 types (true *de novo* and possible *de novo*). True *de novo* disease (when the original disease is known) and possible *de novo* disease (when the original disease is unknown).

De novo disease is classified according to primary structural involvement in the kidney such as glomerular, arterial or interstitium of the kidney. *Table I* shows the classification of *de novo* disease according to the pathophysiologic mechanisms involved. Occurrence of *de novo* renal diseases can be secondary to various reasons such as immunological, metabolic, infectious, and systemic diseases. *Table II* shows the pathophysiologic mechanisms involved in various diseases. The current section illustrates the important immunological and non-immunological glomerular diseases which are seen *de novo* after renal transplantation.

De novo glomerular diseases

Minimal change nephropathy (MCN)

The most uncommon cause of *de novo* disease is MCN. A total of nine cases have been described in the literature [3]. MCN responds well to steroid therapy and graft outcome is good. MCN should be included in the differential diagnosis of post-transplant nephrotic syndrome.

Table I. Classification of *de novo* renal diseases after renal transplantation

- **Immune mediated:**
Minimal change disease
Immunoglobulin A nephropathy
Membranous nephropathy
Membranoproliferative glomerulonephritis
Cresenting glomerulonephritis
Immunotactoid glomerulonephritis
Post-infectious glomerulonephritis

- **Metabolic diabetes:**
Amyloidosis
Light chain disease
Cryoglobulinemia

- **Vascular:**
Hemolytic uremic syndrome/thrombotic thrombocytopenic purpura
Athero-embolic disease

- **Infections:**
Polyoma virus
Bacterial pyelonephritis

Table II. Pathophysiologic mechanisms of various *de novo* diseases

Disease type	Causes	Pathophysiology
FSGS	Chronic allograft nephropathy Virus (Parvovirus B19)	Immunological and non immunological
MPGN	Virus (hepatitis B,G)	Immunological (with and without cryogolobulinemia)
MN	Virus (hepatitis B,C) Tubular injury	Immunological, acute rejection?
ANCA VASCULITIS	?	Immunological
ANTI-GBM (Alport's syndrome)	Defect in type IV collagen	Immunological
HUS/TTP	Medications (cyclosporine, tacrolimus, rapamycin) Virus (CMV, hepatitis)	Immunological
Diabetic nephropathy	Medications (cyclosporine, tacrolimus, steroids) Others (age, obesity)	Hyperglycemia

Focal segmental glomerulosclerosis (FSGS)

De novo FSGS can be seen as a histological finding in many diseases. The differential diagnoses include chronic allograft nephropathy (CAN), various infections and others. Renal transplant recipients with CAN may have histological features of FSGS [4]. Renal grafts with these lesions have poor long-term graft survival. The pathogenesis of FSGS in such cases is similar to CAN (immunological and non-immunological). Various infections have been postulated to induce *de novo* FSGS. Correlation between Parvovirus B19 infection and FSGS has been suggested [5]. Other form of *de novo* FSGS is the collapsing variant and is associated with rapid progression towards graft failure [6]. *De novo* can occur as late as 32 years post-transplantation [7]. The graft survival of *de novo* FSGS remains guarded.

Membranoproliferative glomerulonephritis (MPGN)

MPGN can occur *de novo* after renal transplantation [8-11]. This is associated with hepatitis C infection with or without cryoglobulinemia [8-11]. Hepatitis C related MPGN manifests with proteinuria and is associated with hypocomplementemia [8]. Immunological and virological studies are useful to identify and differentiate this condition from CAN [8].

Membranous nephropathy (MN)

MN is an uncommon form of glomerulonephritis in renal allograft and can be secondary to hepatitis C infections. In a single center series, a total of 15 cases of MN were documented among 409 hepatitis C positive transplant recipients [12]. Two thirds of these were *de novo* and the remaining one third had recurrent MN. The prognosis of MN secondary to hepatitis C is similar to MPGN. *De novo* MN has been associated with numerous foam cells in renal histology [13]. The clinical importance of this lesion remains unclear.

From Renal allograft disease registry (RADR), out of 4,967 renal transplants between 6 centers, only 16 cases of biopsy proven MN have been identified [2]. Ten out of these cases had *de novo* MN as original kidney disease was either different or unknown. From this study, *de novo* MN contributed in 2/3 of the cases. Long-term follow-up was associated with lower graft survival.

The pathophysiologic mechanism of *de novo* MN is synonymous to Heyman nephritis. The release of tubular epithelial antigen into circulation results in deposition of immune complexes in the epimembranous area. Clinical manifestations of this disease is associated with massive proteinuria, progressive renal dysfunction not amenable to any therapy. It is possible that the primary renal injury is due to acute rejection contributing to renal epithelial injury. This results in a cascade of events resulting in *de novo* MN. With the reduction in acute rejection rates, *de novo* MN appears to be a less common problem.

Other glomerulonephritis

Anti-neutrophilic cytoplasmic antibody (ANCA) associated vasculitis has been described occurring *de novo* in renal grafts [14, 15]. The pathophysical mechanics of ANCA associated vasculitis is similar to native kidney vasculitis. *De novo* immunotacturd glomerulopathy has been described with CMV infection [16] and SLE [17] have been implicated.

De novo *crescentic glomerulonephritis in patients with Alport's syndrome*

Asymptomatic *de novo* anti-GBM disease is common in renal grafts of Alport's recipients. However, a small proportion of patients with crescentic glomerulonephritis progress towards irreversible graft failure. Antibodies from Alport recipients are specific to NC1 domain hexamer of type IV collagen. Recipients form antibody to alpha 3 (IV) chain and or the alpha 4 (IV) chain [18]. Patients augment an immune response to foreign protein which is absent in their body due to mutation or deletion of COL4A5 gene. The reason for why certain patients develop significant graft dysfunction is not clear. It has been thought that the difference in the genotypic effect may influence patients developing crescentic glomerulonephritis. Therapy aiming towards inhibiting antibody production by cytotoxic agents (Cytoxan) and elimination of antibody by plasma pheresis have not been successful.

Hemolytic uremic syndrome/thrombotic thrombocytopenic purpura (HUS/TTP)

Occurrence of this disease after transplantation has been associated with significant graft failure [2]. Over the last two decades, immunosuppressive medications such as cyclosporine, tacrolimus and rapamycin have been associated with a higher prevalence of *de novo* HUS/TTP. Approximately 1% of transplant recipients with cyclosporine and rapamycin develop *de novo* HUS/TTP within 1 year follow-up [19]. These patients manifest renal dysfunction with or without proteinuria. The pathophysiology of this disease is thought to be secondary to endothelial injury which may have been mediated by viral infection leading to HUS/TTP. Hepatitis C and CMV infections have been implicated as a causative factor in few cases [20]. There is no specific treatment for this disease. Withdrawal/reduction of offending immunosuppressive medications have been suggested to improve the condition in anecdotal deposits [21].

Other glomerular diseases

With improved long-term success after renal transplant and diabetogenic property of many immunosuppressive agents, *de novo* diabetic nephropathy is becoming a clinical problem [22]. Rare conditions such as light chain nephropathy [23] and amyloidosis [24] can also occur *de novo* in renal grafts.

Conclusion

With improved long-term graft survival after renal transplantation, *de novo* diseases are becoming an important cause for graft dysfunction and failure. Exploring the pathogenesis of individual diseases and optimizing therapy for these diseases remain a challenge for the 21st century.

References

1. Hariharan S. Recurrent and *de novo* diseases after renal transplantation. *Semin Dial* 2000; 13: 195-9.
2. Hariharan S, Adams MB, Brennan DC, et al. Recurrent and *de novo* glomerular disease after renal transplantation: a report from Renal Allograft Disease Registry (RADR). *Transplantation* 1999; 69: 635-41.
3. Markowitz GS, Stemmer CL, Croker BP, D'Agati VD. *De novo* minimal change disease. *Am J Kidney Dis* 1998; 3: 508-13.
4. Cosio FG, Frankel WL, Pelletier RP, Pesavento TE, Henry ML, Ferguson RM. Focal segmental glomerulosclerosis in renal allografts with chronic nephropathy: implications for graft survival. *Am J Kidney Dis* 1999; 34: 731-78.
5. Moudgil A, Nast CC, Bagga A, et al. Association of parvovirus B19 infection with idiopathic collapsing glomerulopathy. *Kidney Int* 2001; 49: 2126-33.
6. Meehan SM, Pascual M, Williams WW, et al. *De novo* collapsing glomerulopathy in renal allografts. *Transplantation* 1998; 65: 1192-7.
7. Trimarchi HM, Gonzalez JM, Truong LD, Brennan TS, Barrios R, Suki WN. Focal segmental Glomerulosclerosis in a 32-year-old kidney allograft after 7 years without immunosuppression. *Nephron* 1999; 82: 270-3.
8. Cruzado JM, Gil-Vernet S, Ercilla G, et al. Hepatitis C virus-associated membranoproliferative glomerulonephritis in renal allografts. *J Am Soc Nephrol* 1996; 7: 2469-75.
9. Morales JM, Campistol JM, Andres A, Rodicio JL. Glomerular diseases in patients with hepatitis C virus infection after renal transplantation. *Curr Opin Nephrol Hypertens* 1997; 6: 511-5.
10. Hammoud H, Haem J, Laurent B, et al. Glomerular disease during HCV infection in renal transplantation. *Nephrol Dial Transplant* 1996; 11: 54-5.
11. Berthoux P, Laurent B, Cecillon S, Berthoux F. Membranoproliferative glomerulonephritis with subendothelial deposits (type I) associated with hepatitis G virus infection in a renal transplant recipient. *Am J Nephrol* 1999; 19: 513-8.
12. Morales JM, Pascual-Capdevila J, Campistol JM, et al. Membranous glomerulonephritis associated with hepatitis C virus infection in renal transplant patients. *Transplantation* 1997; 63: 1634-9.
13. Lal SM, Luger AM, Saha LK, Ross G Jr. *De novo* membranous glomerulopathy in renal allografts with unusual histology. *Int J Artif Organs* 1995; 18: 78-80.
14. Asif A, Toral C, Diego J, Miller J, Roth D. *De novo* ANCA-associated vasculitis occurring 14 years after kidney transplantation. *Am J Kidney Dis* 2000; 35: E10.
15. Schultz DR, Diego JM. Antineutrophil cytoplasmic antibodies (ANCA) and systemic vasculitis: update of assays, immunopathogenesis, controversies and report of a novel *de novo* ANCA-associated vasculitis after kidney transplantation. *Semin Arthritis Rheum* 2000; 29: 267-85.
16. Rao KV, Hafner GP, Crary GS, Andersen WR, Crosson JT. *De novo* immunotactoid glomerulopathy of the renal allograft; possible association with cytomegalovirus infection. *Am J Kidney Dis* 1994; 24: 97-103.
17. Isaac J, Herrara GA, Shihab FS. *De novo* fibrillary glomerulopathy in the renal allograft of a patient with systemic lupus erythematosus. *Nephron* 2001; 87: 365-8.
18. Rutgers A, Meyers KE, Canziani G, Kalluri R, Lin J, Madaio MP. High affinity of anti-GMB antibodies from Goodpasture and transplanted Alport patients to alpha3(IV)NC1 collagen. *Kidney Int* 2000; 58: 115-22.
19. Kahan BD. Efficacy of sirolimus compared with azathioprine for reduction in renal allograft rejection: a randomized multicentre study. The Rapamune US Study Group. *Lancet* 2000; 356: 194-202.
20. Baid S, Pascual M, Williams WW Jr, et al. Renal thrombotic microangiopathy associated with anticardiolipin antibodies in hepatitis C-positive renal allograft recipients. *J Am Soc Nephrol* 1999; 10: 146-53.
21. Hariharan S, Munda R, Cavallo T, et al. Rescue therapy with tacrolimus after combined kidney/pancreas and isolated pancreas transplantation in patients with severe cyclosporine nephrotoxicity. *Transplantation* 1996; 61: 1161-5.
22. Sharma UK, Jha V, Gupta KL, Joshi K, Sakhuja V. *De novo* diabetic glomerulosclerosis in a renal allograft recipient. *Am J Kidney Dis* 1994; 23: 597-9.
23. Ecder T, Tbakhi A, Braun WE, Tubbs RR, Myles J, McMahon JT. *De novo* light-chain deposition disease in a cadaver renal allograft. *Am J Kidney Dis* 1996; 28: 461-5.
24. Le QC, Wood TC, Alpers CE. *De novo* AL amyloid in a renal allograft. *Am J Nephrol* 1998; 18: 67-70.

Recurrent disease in the urological patient following renal transplantation

Guy H. Neild, Christopher R.J. Woodhouse, Susan Wood,
Rohan Nauth-Misir, Senthil Nathan, Niki Jenkins

Institute of Urology and Nephrology, University College London, and Renal Unit UCL Hospitals, London, United Kingdom

Our experience

Background

The Institute of Urology and Nephrology (incorporating the former St Peter's Hospitals) is a tertiary referral centre with a specialist adolescent urology unit. Because of our close links with the Hospital for Sick Children, Great Ormond Street, we follow up many of their patients when they reach adolescence.

These patients, who have end-stage renal failure as a consequence of urological abnormalities, fall into two broad groups: 1) those with "normal" bladders and normal calibre ureters and 2) those with "abnormal" bladders and dilated ureters, or some form of continent or incontinent urinary diversion. Bladder was considered normal if urine flow rate was greater than 15 ml/sec, and there was no residual volume see on ultrasound after voiding.

Since 1.1.85, when cyclosporin was introduced for routine use for all our transplant recipients, up to 1.1.00, we have transplanted 127 urological patients of whom half had normal and half abnormal bladders *(Table I)*. Since 1.4.97 tacrolimus has replaced cyclosporin as our routine calcineurin inhibitor.

Fifty-seven patients with abnormal bladders had 64 transplants, including one patient who had three transplants during this period. The causes of abnormal bladders are shown in *Table II*. Data in *Table II* refer to each transplant. In 47 cases the ureters were transplanted into unaugmented bladder; in the remaining 17 cases there was some form of augmentation or diversion *(Table II)*. Results are compared with 63 transplants in 57 patients, who had renal failure from primary vesico-ureteric reflux or renal dysplasia and whose bladder function was considered to be normal.

Table I. St Peter's experience. Demography

	Abnormal	Normal
Transplant numbers	64	63
Male: female	53:11	31:32
Cyclosporin: tacrolimus	54:10	51:12
Live related	36%	24%
Age-mean (median)	32 (31) years	41 (39) years
Patient number	57	57

Table II. St Peter's experience. Causes of abnormal bladders

Primary pathology		Entero-cystoplasty	Conduit	Continent reservoir
Neuropathic	10 (16%)		3	
Congenital bladder outflow obstruction	43 (67%)	4	3	
Cloacal abnormality	1			1
Exstrophy	3 (5%)		2	1
Renal dysplasia	2			
Prune belly	2			
Tuberculosis	3 (5%)	1	2	

Table III. St Peter's experience. Graft outcome and patient survival

Graft outcome	Abnormal	Normal
1 year	86%	83%
5 year	68%	68%
10 year	59%	60%
15 year	47%	60%
Half-life	16 years	29-33 years
Patient survival	**Abnormal**	**Normal**
1 year	98%	98%
5 year	96%	86%
10 year	88%	86%
15 year	88%	86%

Transplant outcome

There was no difference in actuarial graft survival in the two groups at 10 years with both groups having 60% of grafts functioning, although longer follow-up is showing an advantage for normal bladders with a kidney half-life of 29-33 years compared with 16 years for the abnormal bladders. Similarly actuarial patient survival at 15 years is 86% in both groups *(Table III)*.

Current renal function is better in the group with normal bladders. At latest follow-up, the abnormal, unaugmented bladder group (n = 24) have been followed 93 (76) months [mean (median)] and have a plasma creatinine of 180 (160) µmol/l; whilst the normal bladder group (n = 35) have been followed 84 (75) months and have a creatinine concentration of 154 (131) µmol/l.

We have previously reported that symptomatic urinary tract infections were common in the first 3 months after transplantation (63%); fever and systemic symptoms occurred in 39% with normal bladders and 59% with abnormal bladders. Urinary tract infection directly contributed to graft loss in patients with abnormal bladders, but caused no consequences in those with normal bladders [1, 2].

Discussion

Abnormal native bladders

Despite earlier reports to the contrary [3, 4], recent experience of transplantation in patients with abnormal bladders is very encouraging and similar to our own *(Table IV)* [5-11]. As outcome has improved attention has turned to quality of graft renal function. In a study of 18 children with a 10-year follow-up, mean creatinine was 230 µmol/l and not significantly different form a matched control group similar to our "normal bladder" group [5]. However, in a similar but much larger review of 66 children with PUV, creatinine was similar in the two groups at 7 years (130 µmol/l) but remained stable in controls while it was significantly higher at 10 years in the PUV group (240 µmol/l) [7]. (However, comparing plasma creatinine values in growing adolescents is fairly meaningless).

Table IV. Renal transplantation into abnormal bladders

Diagnosis	Number	Mean age at Tx	5 year graft survival (vs controls)	10 year graft survival (vs controls)	Augmented/ diverted systems	10 year creatinine (vs controls)	Ref.
PUV	18 (paed)	9.1	62% (vs 48)	54% (vs 41)	0	2.3 mg/dl (vs 2.0)	1998 [5]
Urological	18 (paed)	8.4	81%	–	61% augment. 11% conduit	1.4 mg/dl (at 5 yr)	1999 [6]
PUV	66 (paed)	9.4	69% (vs 72)	54% (vs 50)	6%	224 µmol/l (vs 130)	1997 [7]
PUV	23 (adolescent)	16.3	69%	63%	0	1.5 mg/dl (at 7 years)	1995 [8]
PUV	16 (paed)		59%	–	5%	2.0 mg/dl (at 7 years)	1994 [9]
Caeco-cystoplasty	14 (paed)	12.3	84%	73% (censored)	100%	1.4 mg/dl (at 7 years)	1998 [10]
Urological	58 (adult)	30	59%	–	43% conduit 2% augment.	–	1999 [11]
St Peter's	64 (adult)	32	68%	59%	11% augment. 16% conduit	180 µmol/l (vs 154 at 8yrs)	

Paed: paediatric; Tx: transplantation; augment.: entero-cystoplasty).

Adult series report similar data. Ross *et al.* in a study of 16 patients with PUV found that graft function did not decline with time and that graft survival was comparable with other transplant recipients [9]. Graft function in their patients was good with a mean plasma creatinine of approximately 160 µmol/l at 1 year with no decline over the following 7-8 years.

In our experience, patients assessed as having abnormal bladders, of which PUV was the commonest cause, had worse graft function after transplantation when compared with those whose bladder function was assessed as being normal, although graft survival was not significantly different between the 2 groups. The cause of relatively poor graft function in patients with PUV or other causes of poor bladder function is unclear. Many have less than ideal bladder function with high filling and/or voiding pressures and often inadequate bladder emptying. Renal biopsies in patients with deteriorating function have demonstrated multi-focal areas of scarring with extensive tubular atrophy and interstitial fibrosis but little evidence of chronic cellular or vascular rejection. ^{99}Tc-DMSA scanning with tomography has shown multiple small scars in these patients, consistent with a "reflux nephropathy" process rather than chronic rejection [2].

Ileal conduits

Transplants into ileal conduits usually result in good graft function and survival albeit with a high surgical complication rate [11-15]. Our patients with urinary diversions did well initially, but by 5 years half had been lost from recurrent UTI. This is in contrast to the review of our experience from 1977 to 1989 in which we reported 9 transplants into ileal loops which resulted in good function and 67% graft survival at 5 years [13].

Augmented bladders (entero-cystoplasties)

Our five patients with augmented bladders did well initially although renal function was relatively poor. All four kidneys that survived for more than 1 year have developed multiple small scars visible on tomographic DMSA scans and renal biopsy in 3 of them showed no evidence of rejection. This suggests that graft dysfunction is related to poor bladder function in these patients. One patient has now practised double micturition for several years with a subsequent improvement in graft function. If this is not sufficient to empty the bladder, then intermittent self-catherisation is started. The experience of others also indicates that transplantation into the augmented bladder works well provided renal and bladder function are monitored closely [10, 15-17]. In two of our patients with deteriorating function attributed to bladder dysfunction, renal function was stabilised or improved after the bladder problem was treated.

Continent reservoir

Our first patient (1990) with a continent reservoir has done very well (creatinine 110 umol/l) although higher vesical pressures when the bladder was full led to some loss of graft function before this was recognised. Our second patient has had recurrent urinary tract infections that have been difficult to eradicate, although her native kidneys have been removed

There are several case reports of transplantation into continent urinary diversions [18, 19]; these have done well in the short term although long term data is still lacking. Experience with continent diversions draining native kidneys indicates that problems with obstruction and infection are common and require close supervision [20-22].

Summary and recommendations

Pre-operative evaluation

Transplantation into the abnormal lower urinary tract requires careful evaluation and follow-up. Thorough pre-operative assessment of bladder function is essential. All patients with abnormal bladders or reservoir must have a full video cystometrogram, to ensure that the bladder reservoir is large and adequately complaint.

If the bladder is small or has not been used for some time, bladder "cycling" may be required, which involves periodically filling and distending the bladder *via* a suprapubic catheter. A recent study of urodynamics prior to transplantation indicates that poor bladder function as shown by small bladder volumes is a predictor of graft loss even in patients with previously normal bladder function [23]. We did not observe this, although poorer outcome was associated with higher voiding pressures and residual volumes.

Intermittent self-catheterization is safe and effective for a patient with a poor flow rate who fails to empty the bladder. This however is only possible with a normal urethra and a co-operative patient. When this is not practical we would attempt to establish supra-pubic drainage *via* a continent stoma, for example a Mitrofanoff stoma.

If a conduit is to be used, then a loopogram and endoscopy must ensure that it is good condition. We do not remove native kidneys unless they are currently causing recurrent or significant urinary tract infection.

Patients considered to have normal bladders require at least a post-micturition bladder ultrasound examination and urinary flow rate.

Post-operative management

We routinely use double-J ureteric stents for all our transplants. Adequacy of urinary drainage must be assessed frequently, even when renal function seems to be good.

Three months after transplant, when the ureteric stent has been removed, we perform (1) ^{51}Cr-EDTA glomerular filtration rate (GFR), (2) ultrasound of kidney and bladder post micturition, (3) dynamic isotope scan (^{99}Tm-MAG3), and (4) static isotope scan (99Tm - DMSA) as a baseline.

The GFR is repeated at 6 months and then annually. Ultrasound and ^{99}Tm-MAG3 are repeated at 1 year, and then when indicated.

Twenty-four hour urine collections for protein are done at 6 months and then annually, although we now prefer to measure the protein/creatinine ratio on all random urine samples from the outpatient clinic.

If there is renal dysfunction, imaging tests are repeated and, if there is a change from baseline, renal biopsy is performed to exclude an immunological cause of dysfunction. If there is a documented deterioration in renal function in the absence of rejection or cyclosporin toxicity, the DMSA scan is repeated and the bladder reassessed urodynamically.

Complications

Urinary tract infections must be detected and treated early and recurrent infections may require long courses of antibiotics or even removal of the native tracts. All our patients with urological problems receive prophylactic antibiotics for the first six months and continue for longer if a UTI occurs. If urinary tract infections recur, or increase in frequency, then a cause must be sought with ultrasound of kidney and bladder. A plain abdominal X-ray is essential to look for stones in native or transplant kidneys, the bladder, or urinary diversion. If there is a residual volume after double micturition then the patient must be instructed to perform intermittent clean self-catheterization. With these measures good results are obtained.

References

1. Crowe A, Cairns HS, Wood S, Rudge CJ, Woodhouse CR, Neild GH. Renal transplantation following renal failure due to urological disorders. *Nephrol Dial Transplant* 1998; 13: 2065-9.
2. Cairns HS, Spencer S, Hilson AJ, Rudge CJ, Neild GH. 99mTc-DMSA imaging with tomography in renal transplant recipients with abnormal lower urinary tracts. *Nephrol Dial Transplant* 1994; 9: 1157-61.
3. Reinberg Y, Gonzalez R, Fryd D, Mauer SM, Najarian JS. The outcome of renal transplantation in children with posterior urethral valves. *J Urol* 1988; 140: 1491-3.
4. Groenewegen AA, Sukhai RN, Nauta J, Scholtmeyer RJ, Nijman RJ. Results of renal transplantation in boys treated for posterior urethral valves. *J Urol* 1993; 149: 1517-20.
5. Indudhara R, Joseph DB, Perez LM, Diethelm AG. Renal transplantation in children with posterior urethral valves revisited: a 10-year followup. *J Urol* 1998; 160: 1201-3.
6. Koo HP, Bunchman TE, Flynn JT, Punch JD, Schwartz AC, Bloom DA. Renal transplantation in children with severe lower urinary tract dysfunction. *J Urol* 1999; 161: 240-5.
7. Salomon L, Fontaine E, Gagnadoux MF, Broyer M, Beurton D. Posterior urethral valves: long-term renal function consequences after transplantation. *J Urol* 1997; 157: 992-5.
8. Connolly JA, Miller B, Bretan PN. Renal transplantation in patients with posterior urethral valves: favorable long-term outcome. *J Urol* 1995; 154: 1153-5.
9. Ross JH, Kay R, Novick AC, Hayes JM, Hodge EE, B. Long-term results of renal transplantation into the valve bladder. *J Urol* 1994; 151: 1500-4.
10. Fontaine E, Gagnadoux MF, Niaudet P, Broyer M, Beurton D. Renal transplantation in children with augmentation cystoplasty: long-term results. *J Urol* 1998; 159: 2110-3.
11. Akoh JA, Choon TC, Akyol MA, Kyle K, Briggs JD. Outcome of renal transplantation in patients with lower urinary tract abnormality. *J R Coll Surg Edinb* 1999; 44: 78-81.
12. Glass NR, Uehling D, Sollinger H, Belzer F. Renal transplantation using ileal conduits in 5 cases. *J Urol* 1985; 133: 666-8.
13. Cairns HS, Leaker BR, Woodhouse CR, Rudge CJ, Neild GH. Renal transplantation into abnormal lower urinary tract. *Lancet* 1991; 338: 1376-9.
14. Hatch DA, Belitsky P, Barry JM, et al. Fate of renal allografts transplanted in patients with urinary diversions. *Transplantation* 1993; 56: 838-42.
15. Nguyen DH, Reinberg Y, Gonzalez R, Fryd D, Najarian JS. Outcome of renal transplantation after urinary diversion and enterocystoplasty: a retrospective, controlled study. *J Urol* 1990; 144: 1349-51.

16. Thomalla JV. Augmentation of the bladder in preparation for renal transplantation. *Surg Gynecol Obstet* 1990; 170: 349-52.
17. Zaragoza MR, Ritchey ML, Bloom DA, McGuire EJ. Enterocystoplasty in renal transplantation candidates: urodynamic evaluation and outcome. *J Urol* 1993; 150: 1463-6.
18. Marechal JM, Sanseverino R, Gelet A, Martin X, Salas M, Dubernard JM. Continent cutaneous ileostomy (Kock Pouch) prior to renal transplantation. *Br J Urol* 1990; 65: 317-21.
19. Hatch DA. Kidney transplantation in patients with an abnormal lower urinary tract. *Urol Clin North Am* 1994; 21: 311-20.
20. Hensle TW, Connor JP, Burbige KA. Continent urinary diversion in childhood. *J Urol* 1990; 143: 981-3.
21. Cendron M, Gearhart JP. The Mitrofanoff principle: Technique and application in continent urinary diversion. *Urol Clin North Am* 1991; 18: 615-21.
22. Woodhouse CR, Gordon EM. The Mitrofanoff principle for urethral failure. *Br J Urol* 1994; 73: 55-60.
23. Kashi SH, Wynne KS, Sadek SA, Lodge JP. An evaluation of vesical urodynamics before renal transplantation and its effect on renal allograft function and survival. *Transplantation* 1994; 57: 1455-7.

Achevé d'imprimer par Corlet, Imprimeur, S.A.
14110 Condé-sur-Noireau (France)
N° d'Imprimeur : 3403 - Dépôt légal : novembre 2001
Imprimé en U.E.